Valvular Heart Disease and Heart Failure

Editors

JYOTHY J. PUTHUMANA
RAGAVENDRA R. BALIGA

HEART FAILURE CLINICS

www.heartfailure.theclinics.com

Consulting Editor
EDUARDO BOSSONE

Founding Editor
JAGAT NARULA

July 2023 • Volume 19 • Number 3

ELSEVIER

1600 John F. Kennedy Boulevard • Suite 1800 • Philadelphia, Pennsylvania, 19103-2899

http://www.theclinics.com

HEART FAILURE CLINICS Volume 19, Number 3
July 2023 ISSN 1551-7136, ISBN-13: 978-0-323-93889-1

Editor: Joanna Gascoine
Developmental Editor: Jessica Cañaberal

Heart Failure Clinics (ISSN 1551-7136) is published quarterly by Elsevier Inc., 360 Park Avenue South, New York, NY 10010-1710. Months of publication are January, April, July, and October. Business and editorial offices: 1600 John F. Kennedy Boulevard, Suite 1800, Philadelphia, PA 19103-2899. Periodicals postage paid at New York, NY, and additional mailing offices. Subscription prices are USD 291.00 per year for US individuals, USD 629.00 per year for US institutions, USD 100.00 per year for US students and residents, USD 315.00 per year for Canadian individuals, USD 729.00 per year for Canadian institutions, USD 331.00 per year for international individuals, USD 729.00 per year for international institutions, and USD 100.00 per year for Canadian and foreign students/residents. To receive student and resident rate, orders must be accompanied by name of affiliated institution, date of term, and the *signature* of program/residency coordinator on institution letterhead. Orders will be billed at individual rate until proof of status is received. Foreign air speed delivery is included in all *Clinics* subscription prices. All prices are subject to change without notice. **POSTMASTER:** Send address changes to *Heart Failure Clinics*, Elsevier Health Sciences Division, Subscription Customer Service, 3251 Riverport Lane, Maryland Heights, MO 63043. **Customer Service: 1-800-654-2452 (US and Canada). From outside of the US and Canada, call 314-447-8871. Fax: 314-447-8029. For print support, E-mail: JournalsCustomerService-usa@elsevier.com. For online support, E-mail: JournalsOnlineSupport-usa@elsevier.com.**

Reprints. For copies of 100 or more of articles in this publication, please contact the Commercial Reprints Department, Elsevier Inc., 360 Park Avenue South, New York, NY 10010-1710. Tel.: 212-633-3874; Fax: 212-633-3820; E-mail: reprints@elsevier.com.

Heart Failure Clinics is covered in *MEDLINE/PubMed (Index Medicus)*.

Contributors

CONSULTING EDITOR

EDUARDO BOSSONE, MD, PhD, FCCP, FESC, FACC
Consulting Editor, *Heart Failure Clinics*,
Director of Cardiology, Cardarelli Hospital,
Naples, Italy

EDITORS

JYOTHY J. PUTHUMANA, MD, FACC, FASE
Associate Professor, Division of Cardiology,
Department of Medicine, Northwestern
Medicine, Northwestern University Feinberg
School of Medicine, Chicago, Illinois, USA

RAGAVENDRA R. BALIGA, MD, MBA, FACP, FRCP (Edin), FACC
Inaugural Cardio-Oncologist Professor and
Attending Cardiologist, Division of Cardiology,
The Ohio State University Wexner Medical
Center, Columbus, Ohio, USA

AUTHORS

FARAZ S. AHMAD, MD, MS
Assistant Professor of Medicine (Cardiology),
Division of Cardiology, Department of
Medicine, Bluhm Cardiovascular Institute
Center for Artificial Intelligence, Northwestern
Medicine, Division of Health and Biomedical
Informatics, Department of Preventive
Medicine, Northwestern University Feinberg
School of Medicine, Chicago, Illinois,
USA

VINESH APPADURAI, MBBS
Bluhm Cardiovascular Institute, Northwestern
University, Chicago, Illinois, USA; School of
Medicine, The University of Queensland,
St Lucia, Australia

GLORIA AYUBA, DO
Bluhm Cardiovascular Institute, Northwestern
University, Chicago, Illinois, USA

PHILIPPE B. BERTRAND, MD, PhD
Faculty of Medicine and Life Sciences, Hasselt
University, Diepenbeek, Belgium; Department of
Cardiology, Hospital Oost-Limburg Genk, Genk,
Belgium

ROBERT O. BONOW, MD, MS
Division of Cardiology, Northwestern University
Feinberg School of Medicine, Chicago, Illinois,
USA

KHADIJAH BREATHETT, MD, MS, FACC, FAHA, FHFSA
Tenured Associate Professor of Medicine,
Division of Cardiovascular Medicine, Krannert
Cardiovascular Research Center, Indiana
University, Indianapolis, Indiana, USA

CAROLINE CANNING, MSc, MBI
Division of Cardiology, Department of
Medicine, Northwestern University Feinberg
School of Medicine, Bluhm Cardiovascular
Institute Center for Artificial Intelligence,
Northwestern Medicine, Chicago, Illinois, USA

MARIE-ANNICK CLAVEL, DVM, PhD
Institut Universitaire de Cardiologie et de
Pneumologie de Québec, Université Laval
(IUCPQ-UL)/Québec Heart and Lung Institute,
Laval University, Québec City, Québec,
Canada; Department of Cardiology, Odense
University Hospital, University of Southern
Denmark, Odense, Denmark

CHARLES J. DAVIDSON, MD
Northwestern University Feinberg School of Medicine, Chicago, Illinois, USA

SÉBASTIEN DEFERM, MD, PhD
Faculty of Medicine and Life Sciences, Hasselt University, Diepenbeek, Belgium; Department of Cardiology, Mainz University Hospital, Mainz, Germany

AKSHAY S. DESAI, MD, MPH
Medical Director, Cardiomyopathy and Heart Failure Program, Department of Cardiology, Brigham and Women's Hospital, Associate Professor, Harvard Medical School, Boston, Massachusetts, USA

SEBASTIAAN DHONT, MD
Faculty of Medicine and Life Sciences, Hasselt University, Diepenbeek, Belgium; Department of Cardiology, Hospital Oost-Limburg Genk, Genk, Belgium

KENDALL FREE, BS
Graduate Student, Department of Biofunction Research, Tokyo Medical and Dental University, Tokyo, Japan

MUHAMMED GERÇEK, MD
Clinic for General and Interventional Cardiology/Angiology, Heart and Diabetes Center NRW, Ruhr University Bochum, Bad Oeynhausen, Germany; Northwestern University, Feinberg School of Medicine, Chicago, Illinois, USA

JAMES GUO
Division of Cardiology, Department of Medicine, Northwestern University Feinberg School of Medicine, Bluhm Cardiovascular Institute Center for Artificial Intelligence, Northwestern Medicine, Chicago, Illinois, USA

REBECCA T. HAHN, MD
Department of Medicine, Columbia University Medical Center/NewYork-Presbyterian Hospital, New York, USA

ONYEDIKA ILONZE, MD, MPH, FACC, FHFSA
Assistant Professor of Clinical Medicine, Division of Cardiovascular Medicine, Krannert Cardiovascular Research Center, Indiana University, Indianapolis, Indiana, USA

GUILLAUME JEAN, MD
Institut Universitaire de Cardiologie et de Pneumologie de Québec, Université Laval (IUCPQ-UL)/Québec Heart and Lung Institute, Laval University, Québec City, Québec, Canada

MARK A. LEBEHN, MD
Department of Medicine, Columbia University Medical Center/NewYork-Presbyterian Hospital, New York, USA

SABRA LEWSEY, MD, MPH, FACC
Assistant Professor of Medicine, Division of Cardiology, Department of Medicine, Johns Hopkins School of Medicine, Baltimore, Maryland, USA

AMRIT MISRA, MD
Adult Congenital Heart Disease Fellow, Department of Cardiology, Boston Chidren's Hospital, Department of Medicine, Division of Cardiology, Brigham and Women's Hospital, Harvard Medical School, Boston, Massachusetts, USA

NILS SOFUS BORG MOGENSEN, MD
Institut Universitaire de Cardiologie et de Pneumologie de Québec, Université Laval (IUCPQ-UL)/Québec Heart and Lung Institute, Laval University, Québec City, Québec, Canada; Department of Cardiology, Odense University Hospital, University of Southern Denmark, Odense, Denmark

AKHIL NARANG, MD
Assistant Professor of Medicine (Cardiology), Division of Cardiology, Department of Medicine, Northwestern University Feinberg School of Medicine, Bluhm Cardiovascular Institute Center for Artificial Intelligence, Northwestern Medicine, Chicago, Illinois, USA

GRAHAM PEIGH, MD, MSc
Division of Cardiology, Northwestern University Feinberg School of Medicine, Chicago, Illinois, USA

JYOTHY J. PUTHUMANA, MD, FACC, FASE
Associate Professor, Division of Cardiology, Department of Medicine, Northwestern Medicine, Northwestern University Feinberg School of Medicine, Chicago, Illinois, USA

VOLKER RUDOLPH, MD
Clinic for General and Interventional
Cardiology/Angiology, Heart and Diabetes
Center NRW, Ruhr University Bochum, Bad
Oeynhausen, Germany

TAIMUR SAFDUR, MD
Bluhm Cardiovascular Institute, Northwestern
University, Chicago, Illinois, USA

ALEXANDER SHINNERL, BA
Medical School Student, College of Medicine,
Indiana University, Indianapolis, Indiana, USA

BRODY SLOSTAD, MD
Bluhm Cardiovascular Institute, Northwestern
University, Chicago, Illinois, USA

JAMES D. THOMAS, MD
Professor of Medicine (Cardiology),
Division of Cardiology, Department of
Medicine, Northwestern University Feinberg
School of Medicine, Bluhm Cardiovascular

Institute Center for Artificial Intelligence,
Northwestern Medicine, Chicago, Illinois,
USA

ANNE MARIE VALENTE, MD
Director, Boston Adult Congenital
Heart Program, Department of Cardiology,
Boston Children's Hospital, Department of
Medicine, Division of Cardiology, Brigham
and Women's Hospital, Professor, Harvard
Medical School, Boston, Massachusetts,
USA

PIETER M. VANDERVOORT, MD
Faculty of Medicine and Life Sciences, Hasselt
University, Diepenbeek, Belgium; Department
of Cardiology, Hospital Oost-Limburg Genk,
Genk, Belgium

RALPH S. VON BARDELEBEN, MD
Department of Cardiology, Mainz University
Hospital, Mainz, Germany

Contents

Preface: Monitoring for Valve Decrepitude: Surveillance Echo for All at Age 60…?   xi

Jyothy J. Puthumana, Ragavendra R. Baliga, and Eduardo Bossone

Aortic Valvular Stenosis and Heart Failure: Advances in Diagnostic, Management, and Intervention   273

Guillaume Jean, Nils Sofus Borg Mogensen, and Marie-Annick Clavel

Up to 30% of patients with aortic stenosis (AS) present with heart failure (HF) symptoms with either reduced or preserved left ventricular ejection fraction. Many of these patients present with a low-flow state, reduced aortic-valve-area (≤ 1.0 cm^2) with low aortic-mean-gradient and aortic-peak-velocity (<40 mm Hg and <4.0 m/s). Thus, determination of true severity is essential for correct management, and multi-imaging evaluation must be performed. Medical treatment of HF is imperative and should be optimized concurrently with the determination of AS-severity. Finally, AS should be treated according to guidelines, keeping in mind that HF and low-flow increase interventions risks.

Aortic Regurgitation and Heart Failure: Advances in Diagnosis, Management, and Interventions   285

Graham Peigh, Jyothy J. Puthumana, and Robert O. Bonow

This review discusses the contemporary clinical evaluation and management of patients with comorbid aortic regurgitation (AR) and heart failure (HF) (AR-HF). Importantly, as clinical HF exists along the spectrum of AR severity, the present review also details novel strategies to detect early signs of HF before the clinical syndrome ensues. Indeed, there may be a vulnerable cohort of AR patients who benefit from early detection and management of HF. Additionally, while the mainstay of operative management for AR has historically been surgical aortic valve replacement, this review discusses alternate procedures that may be beneficial in high-risk cohorts.

Primary Mitral Regurgitation and Heart Failure: Current Advances in Diagnosis and Management   297

Brody Slostad, Gloria Ayuba, and Jyothy J. Puthumana

Primary mitral regurgitation is a frequent etiology of congestive heart failure and is best treated with intervention when patients are symptomatic or when additional risk factors exist. Surgical intervention improves outcomes in appropriately selected patients. However, for those at high surgical risk, transcatheter intervention provides less invasive repair and replacement options while providing comparable outcomes to surgery. The excess mortality and high prevalence of heart failure in untreated mitral regurgitation illuminate the need for further developments in mitral valve intervention ideally fulfilled by expanding these types of procedures and eligibility to these procedures beyond only those at high surgical risk.

Secondary Mitral Regurgitation and Heart Failure: Current Advances in Diagnosis and Management   307

Muhammed Gerçek, Akhil Narang, Jyothy J. Puthumana, Charles J. Davidson, and Volker Rudolph

> The causes of mitral regurgitation (MR) can be broadly divided into primary and secondary causes. Although primary MR is caused by degenerative alterations of the mitral valve and the mitral valve apparatus, secondary (functional) MR is multifactorial and related to dilation of the left ventricle and/or mitral annulus commonly resulting in concomitant restriction of the leaflets. Therefore, the treatment of secondary MR (SMR) is complex and includes guideline directed heart failure therapy along with surgical and transcatheter approaches that have shown effectiveness in certain subgroups. This review aims to provide insight into current advances in diagnosis and management of SMR.

Assessment of Right Ventricle Function and Tricuspid Regurgitation in Heart Failure: Current Advances in Diagnosis and Imaging   317

Vinesh Appadurai, Taimur Safdur, and Akhil Narang

 Video content accompanies this article at http://www.heartfailure.theclinics.com.

> Right ventricular (RV) systolic dysfunction increases mortality among heart failure patients, and therefore, accurate diagnosis and monitoring is paramount. RV anatomy and function are complex, usually requiring a combination of imaging modalities to completely quantitate volumes and function. Tricuspid regurgitation usually occurs with RV dysfunction, and quantifying this valvular lesion also may require multiple imaging modalities. Echocardiography is the first-line imaging tool for identifying RV dysfunction, with cardiac MRI and cardiac computed tomography adding valuable additional information.

Valvular Heart Failure due to Tricuspid Regurgitation: Surgical and Transcatheter Management Options   329

Mark A. Lebehn and Rebecca T. Hahn

 Video content accompanies this article at http://www.heartfailure.theclinics.com.

> Given the independent association of mortality with higher grades of tricuspid regurgitation severity, there is an increasing interest in improving the outcomes of this prevalent valvular heart disease. A new classification of tricuspid regurgitation etiology allows for an improved understanding of different pathophysiologic forms of the disease, which may determine the appropriate management strategy. Current surgical outcomes remain suboptimal and multiple transcatheter device therapies are currently under investigation to give high and prohibitive surgical risk patients treatment options beyond medical therapy.

Valvular Regurgitation in Adults with Congenital Heart Disease and Heart Failure: Current Status and Potential Interventions   345

Amrit Misra, Akshay S. Desai, and Anne Marie Valente

> The great majority of patients born with congenital heart disease (CHD) are living well into adulthood, yet they often have residual hemodynamic lesions, including valvar regurgitation. As these complex patients grow older, they are at risk of developing heart failure, which can be exacerbated by the underlying valvular regurgitation. In this review, we describe the etiologies of heart failure related to valvular regurgitation in the CHD population and discuss potential interventions.

Arrythmia-Mediated Valvular Heart Disease   357

Sébastien Deferm, Philippe B. Bertrand, Sebastiaan D'hont, Ralph S. von Bardeleben, and Pieter M. Vandervoort

The aging population is rising at record pace worldwide. Along with it, a steep increase in the prevalence of atrial fibrillation and heart failure with preserved ejection fraction is to be expected. Similarly, both atrial functional mitral and tricuspid regurgitation (AFMR and AFTR) are increasingly observed in daily clinical practice. This article summarizes all current evidence regarding the epidemiology, prognosis, pathophysiology, and therapeutic options. Specific attention is addressed to discern AFMR and AFTR from their ventricular counterparts, given their different pathophysiology and therapeutic needs.

Racial, Ethnic, and Gender Disparities in Valvular Heart Failure Management   379

Onyedika Ilonze, Kendall Free, Alexander Shinnerl, Sabra Lewsey, and Khadijah Breathett

Racial, ethnic, and gender disparities are present in the diagnosis and management of valvular heart disease. The prevalence of valvular heart disease varies by race, ethnicity, and gender, but diagnostic evaluations are not equitable across the groups, which makes the true prevalence less clear. The delivery of evidence-based treatments for valvular heart disease is not equitable. This article focuses on the epidemiology of valvular heart diseases associated with heart failure and the related disparities in treatment, with a focus on how to improve delivery of nonpharmacological and pharmacological treatments.

The Emerging Role of Artificial Intelligence in Valvular Heart Disease   391

Caroline Canning, James Guo, Akhil Narang, James D. Thomas, and Faraz S. Ahmad

Valvular heart disease (VHD) is a morbid condition in which timely identification and evidence-based treatments can lead to improved outcomes. Artificial intelligence broadly refers to the ability for computers to perform tasks and problem solve like the human mind. Studies applying AI to VHD have used a variety of structured (eg, sociodemographic, clinical) and unstructured (eg, electrocardiogram, phonocardiogram, and echocardiograms) and machine learning modeling approaches. Additional researches in diverse populations, including prospective clinical trials, are needed to evaluate the effectiveness and value of AI-enabled medical technologies in clinical care for patients with VHD.

HEART FAILURE CLINICS

FORTHCOMING ISSUES

October 2023
Changing Landscape of Heart Failure Imaging
Purvi Parwani, *Editor*

January 2024
Novel Non-pharmacological Approaches to Heart Failure
Vijay Rao and Geetha Bhat, *Editors*

April 2024
Adult Congenital Heart Disease
Saurabh Rajpal and Ragavendra Baliga, *Editors*

RECENT ISSUES

April 2023
Covid-19
Timothy D. Henry and Santiago Garcia, *Editors*

January 2023
Challenges in Pulmonary Hypertension
Alberto M. Marra, Pietro Ameri, and Alexander Sherman, *Editors*

October 2022
SGLT-2 Inhibitors
Ragavendra R. Baliga and Deepak L. Bhatt, *Editors*

SERIES OF RELATED INTEREST

Cardiology Clinics
http://www.cardiology.theclinics.com/
Cardiac Electrophysiology Clinics
https://www.cardiacep.theclinics.com/
Interventional Cardiology Clinics
https://www.interventional.theclinics.com/

THE CLINICS ARE AVAILABLE ONLINE!
Access your subscription at:
www.theclinics.com

Preface

Monitoring for Valve Decrepitude: Surveillance Echo for All at Age 60…?

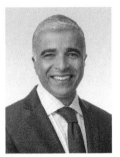
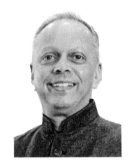
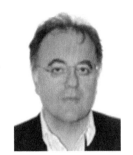

Jyothy J. Puthumana, MD, FACC, FASE

Ragavendra R. Baliga, MD, MBA, FACP, FRCP (Edin), FACC

Eduardo Bossone, MD, PhD, FCCP, FESC, FACC

Editors

BACKGROUND

Heart failure is usually the end point with progression of most valvular lesions, leading to stages B, C, and D heart failure usually preceded by long latent asymptomatic periods. With progression, most valve lesions lead to volume or pressure overload, leading to symptoms of heart failure: fatigue, shortness of breath, early satiety, symptoms and signs related to systemic venous hypertension. Given increased life expectancy across the world, more so in the West, advanced valvular lesion as a cause for symptomatic heart failure has increased, with a significant increase in prevalence beyond the age of 75 years.[1] In a landmark paper from a combination of large epidemiologic studies in the general population from the United States that included comprehensive echocardiographic evaluation of valvular function, moderate or severe valve disease was thought to be present in nearly one in eight subjects (13.3%) aged 75 years and older, with a male predominance. Mitral regurgitation (MR) was the most common lesion followed by aortic stenosis (AS), with most of these subjects having echocardiographic findings of pressure or volume overload, which independently contributed to subsequent mortality.[1–4] This further highlighted the underdiagnosis of severe valve disease in the community and the integral role of quantitative echocardiography in this population. In addition, significant burden of atrial fibrillation in this age group has been independently shown to increase the long-term risk for significant mitral and tricuspid regurgitation,[5] suggesting the need for closer follow-up in this subgroup of elderly patients. There is also increased recognition of delayed diagnosis and treatment among women[6] and other ethnic minorities with recent literature highlighting potential ways to overcome these gaps in care.[7]

Survival of patients with severe valve disease was 79% at 5 years compared with 93% in those without. Furthermore, heart failure was seen in about 64% of patients within 5 years of follow-up among patients with significant MR[8] even in those subjects with left ventricular ejection fraction greater than 50%. Many of these patients are denied intervention despite definite guideline-based indications, mostly because of older age,[9] thereby limiting their symptom-free period before the end of life (**Fig. 1**).

CURRENT EVIDENCE-BASED TREATMENT OPTIONS

The prevalence of heart failure from several studies and registries among patients with severe

Heart Failure Clin 19 (2023) xi–xiv
https://doi.org/10.1016/j.hfc.2023.03.003
1551-7136/23/© 2023 Published by Elsevier Inc.

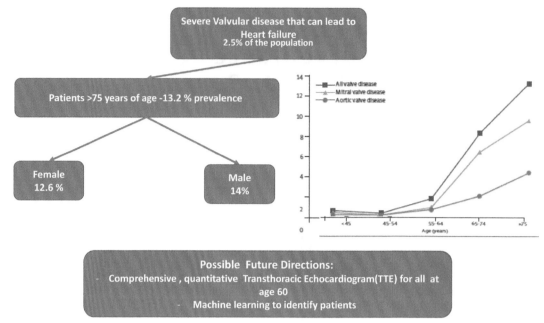

Fig. 1. Prevalence and future directions. (*Reprinted with permission from* Elsevier. The Lancet, September 2006, 368 (9540), 1005-1011.)

AS varies between 10% and 35%. Transcatheter aortic valve replacement (TAVR), initially tested in the high-risk patient and then in intermediate- and low-risk patients, has revolutionized treatment for AS. TAVR even among extremely high-risk patients with decreased ejection fraction was shown to offer significant improvement in survival, lack of progression to heart failure, and an improvement in ejection fraction during follow-up.[10,11] Continued advancement of TAVR technology has pushed the boundaries further regarding timing of intervention, treatment of aortic insufficiency, intervention for bioprosthetic valve degeneration with a TAVR valve in valve, and others.

With recognition of higher prevalence of significant mitral valve regurgitation in the aging population related to ischemic heart disease, fibroelastic degeneration of the leaflets, chronic atrial fibrillation, and similar, research and development in nonsurgical options for mitral valve repair/replacement has seen a rapid growth. This has led to approval of transcatheter edge-to-edge repair (TEER) for the treatment of degenerative MR in the high-risk population, with additional data from the registries suggesting benefits of earlier intervention due to the lower risk of these procedures and the short- and long-term benefits from improved functional status, and decreased risk of progression to heart failure in these patients. Secondary/functional mitral regurgitation (FMR) now

has proven data from the landmark COAPT study showing superiority of TEER compared with maximal continued medical management,[12] the subgroup in whom surgical mitral valve replacement/repair showed no short- or long-term benefits. In addition to approval of TEER in high-risk degenerative MR and FMR, ongoing studies comparing surgical mitral valve repair with TEER in intermediate- (REPAIR-MR) and low-risk (PRIMARY-MR) cohorts will advance the field further.

These studies and other similar ones have mainly contributed to a significant increase in investment, research, and development in the structural heart arena for management of other valvular conditions leading to heart failure.[2,13] Clinically severe tricuspid regurgitation causes long-term morbidity and mortality with a very small subgroup of patients who are eligible by guideline criteria for surgical repair/replacement of the tricuspid valve. Multiple catheter-based interventions in the tricuspid arena have undergone development over the past 10 to 12 years targeting the valve, annulus, coaptation gap, and others, with many currently undergoing early feasibility studies, and one completed pivotal trial (TRILUMINATE) showing definitive improvement in severity of tricuspid regurgitation, functional class, and decreased hospitalizations in the short term. Longer-term follow-up, including its potential impact on long-term survival, is awaited.[13]

In parallel, newer imaging tools in echocardiography, including 3D imaging, automated quantification, tools for detailed evaluation of the valve and annular anatomy and strain imaging have significantly improved understanding of the valvular lesions with better ability to predict appropriate management strategies in these patients. Improved CT and MRI scanners and techniques have also contributed and complemented the ability for more specific thresholds for intervention. These tools have been shown to identify the time point at which the benefit of an intervention for the valvular lesion far exceeds the risk of continued watchful waiting.

FUTURE DIRECTIONS AND OPPORTUNITIES

Further research will help to identify strategies and protocols for effective and efficient use of comprehensive quantitative echocardiography as the gatekeeper given the knowledge of high prevalence, morbidity, and mortality associated with these advanced valvular lesions, especially in the elderly patient and specifically among women. To this end, a high-quality transthoracic echocardiogram done by a well-trained sonographer using contemporary equipment and with the skill set to acquire comprehensive Doppler, adequate 3D data sets, to use currently available automated quantification tools, strain imaging, and thorough quantitative evaluation of the valve lesion and interpreted by an echocardiographer with expertise in valvular disease will help lead to appropriate identification, referral, follow-up, and management of these patients. A screening handheld POCUS (point-of-care ultrasound) will not be able to adequately do justice in this situation. These advancements will enable to identify the appropriate patient, fine-tune the threshold and timing of intervention, and be able to predict the right intervention for the individual patient.

Machine learning has been suggested as a strategy for large-scale identification of cardiovascular pathologic condition from electronic medical records and imaging studies.[14] Similar strategies in large populations among the elderly may help with early identification of significant valvular lesions during the presymptomatic latent period, and those patients could then benefit from a comprehensive transthoracic echocardiogram for further risk stratification and management.

We are fortunate and thankful to have leaders in the field of clinical valvular heart disease, valvular research, diagnostic imaging, structural imaging, adult congenital heart disease, disparities in health care access, and artificial intelligence who have contributed and enriched this issue of the journal on valvular heart disease and heart failure.

Jyothy J. Puthumana, MD, FACC, FASE
Division of Cardiology
Department of Medicine
Northwestern Medicine
Feinberg School of Medicine
676 North St. Clair Street
Chicago, IL 60611, USA

Ragavendra R. Baliga, MD, MBA, FACP, FRCP
(Edin), FACC
Division of Cardiology
The Ohio State University
Wexner Medical Center
Columbus, OH, USA

Eduardo Bossone, MD, PhD, FCCP, FESC, FACC
Cardarelli Hospital
Naples, Italy

E-mail addresses:
jputhuma@nm.org (J.J. Puthumana)
rrbaliga@gmail.com (R.R. Baliga)
ebossone@hotmail.com (E. Bossone)

REFERENCES

1. Nkomo VT, Gardin JM, Skelton TN, et al. Burden of valvular heart diseases: a population-based study. Lancet 2006;368(9540):1005–11.
2. Writing Committee M, Otto CM, Nishimura RA, et al. 2020 ACC/AHA guideline for the management of patients with valvular heart disease: executive summary: a report of the American College of Cardiology/American Heart Association Joint Committee on Clinical Practice Guidelines. J Am Coll Cardiol 2021;77(4):450–500.
3. Supino PG, Borer JS, Preibisz J, et al. The epidemiology of valvular heart disease: a growing public health problem. Heart Fail Clin 2006;2(4):379–93.
4. Vahanian A, Beyersdorf F, Praz F, et al. 2021 ESC/EACTS guidelines for the management of valvular heart disease. Eur Heart J 2022;43(7):561–632.
5. Deferm S, Dauw J, Vandervoort PM, et al. Atrial functional mitral and tricuspid regurgitation. Curr Treat Options Cardio Med 2020;22(10):30.
6. Kislitsina ON, Zareba KM, Bonow RO, et al. Is mitral valve disease treated differently in men and women? Eur J Prev Cardiol 2019;26(13):1433–43.
7. Lewsey SC, Breathett K. Racial and ethnic disparities in heart failure: current state and future directions. Curr Opin Cardiol 2021;36(3):320–8.
8. Dziadzko V, Clavel MA, Dziadzko M, et al. Outcome and undertreatment of mitral regurgitation: a community cohort study. Lancet 2018;391(10124): 960–9.

9. Otto CM, Nishimura RA, Bonow RO, et al. 2020 ACC/AHA guideline for the management of patients with valvular heart disease: a report of the American College of Cardiology/American Heart Association Joint Committee on Clinical Practice Guidelines. Circulation 2021;143(5):e72–227.

10. Dauerman HL, Reardon MJ, Popma JJ, et al. Early recovery of left ventricular systolic function after corevalve transcatheter aortic valve replacement. Circ Cardiovasc Interv 2016;9(6):e003425.

11. Elmariah S, Palacios IF, McAndrew T, et al. Outcomes of transcatheter and surgical aortic valve replacement in high-risk patients with aortic stenosis and left ventricular dysfunction: results from the Placement of Aortic Transcatheter Valves (PARTNER) trial (cohort A). Circ Cardiovasc Interv 2013;6(6):604–14.

12. Stone GW, Lindenfeld J, Abraham WT, et al. Transcatheter mitral-valve repair in patients with heart failure. N Engl J Med 2018;379(24):2307–18.

13. Davidson LJ, Davidson CJ. Transcatheter treatment of valvular heart disease: a review. JAMA 2021;325(24):2480–94.

14. Ahmad FS, Luo Y, Wehbe RM, et al. Advances in machine learning approaches to heart failure with preserved ejection fraction. Heart Fail Clin 2022;18(2):287–300.

Aortic Valvular Stenosis and Heart Failure
Advances in Diagnostic, Management, and Intervention

Guillaume Jean, MD[a], Nils Sofus Borg Mogensen, MD[a,b],
Marie-Annick Clavel, DVM, PhD[a,b],*

KEYWORDS

- Aortic stenosis • Heart failure • Left ventricular ejection fraction • Echocardiography
- Computed tomography

KEY POINTS

- Concomitance of aortic stenosis and heart failure is not an uncommon occurrence, and requires thorough examination to determine the causal relationship between the 2 ailments.
- Patients with heart failure and aortic stenosis can present themselves with discordant echocardiographic findings, making determination of severity of aortic stenosis challenging.
- Determination aortic stenosis severity in patients with discordant echocardiographic findings relies on Dobutamine stress echocardiography and determination of aortic valve calcification by cardiac multidetector computer tomography.

INTRODUCTION

The comprehension and evaluation of aortic stenosis (AS) has advanced significantly in the last decades. At the same time, new intervention methods has evolved greatly but there are still some challenging aspects, especially when AS is present in the setting of heart failure (HF) symptoms, both in patients with reduced (HFrEF) or preserved (HFpEF) left ventricular ejection fraction (LVEF; **Figs. 1** and **2**).

The prevalence of AS increases with age, and 13% of patients aged older than 75 years is estimated to have moderate-to-severe AS.[1] In patients with severe AS, the development of symptoms is associated with worse outcome and higher mortality.[2] As such, AS is the most common valvulopathy referred for surgical management. In North America, AS is estimated to be responsible for more than 150,000 valve replacement and 20,000 deaths, each year.[3,4] In recent years, the management of AS has improved greatly with the possibility of transcatheter aortic-valve replacement as an alternate treatment to surgical aortic valve replacement (SAVR), especially in patient with high and intermediate surgical risk.[5]

Almost one-third of patients with HF symptoms and AS will present with discordant echocardiographic grading—small aortic valve area (AVA) but with low aortic mean gradient and peak velocity, making the assessment of AS-severity uncertain. Such discordant measurements are most often related to reduced flow status and stroke volume.[6] Furthermore, new research indicates that even moderate AS is associated with increased mortality in patients with HF.[7]

[a] Institut Universitaire de Cardiologie et de Pneumologie de Québec, Université Laval (IUCPQ-UL)/ Québec Heart & Lung Institute, Laval University, 2725 Chemin Sainte-Foy, Québec City, QC G1V 4G5, Canada;
[b] Department of Cardiology, Odense University Hospital, University of Southern Denmark, J. B. Winsløws Vej 4, 5000 Odense, Denmark
* Corresponding author. Inst.itut Universitaire de Cardiologie et de Pneumologie de Québec - Laval University, 2725 Chemin Sainte-Foy A-2047, Québec City, QC G1V 4G5, Canada.
E-mail address: marie-annick.clavel@criucpq.ulaval.ca

Heart Failure Clin 19 (2023) 273–283
https://doi.org/10.1016/j.hfc.2023.02.005

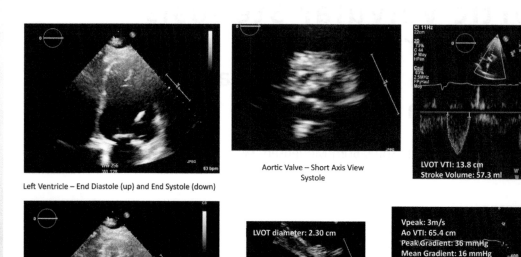

Fig. 1. Echocardiographic examination of a patient with aortic stenosis and reduced ejection fraction. Ao, aorta; AVA, aortic valve area; LVOT, left ventricular outflow tract; Vpeak, peak aortic jet velocity; VTI, velocity-time integral.

In this article, we will review the pathophysiology of the concomitance of HF and AS, the different diagnostic modalities and criterions for the assessment of AS-severity, and the indication of treatment in patients with concomitant HF and AS.

Pathophysiology and Etiology of Aortic Stenosis and Its Association with Heart Failure

Both congenital and acquired causes are associated with the development of AS. The most prevalent congenital cause is bicuspid aortic valve but also includes unicuspid and quadricuspid aortic valve or subaortic obstruction.[8] Acquired causes for AS are more heterogeneous. Worldwide, the most common cause for AS is rheumatic valve disease but in industrialized countries, degenerative valve disease is the most prevalent cause of AS. The exact mechanisms leading to degeneration is not yet fully understood but the development of AS is associated with traditional cardiovascular risk factors; diabetes, high cholesterol, high blood pressure, chronic renal failure, and most importantly age.[9]

Degenerative or calcific AS is caused by shear stress in the valve, leading to thickening and calcification of the leaflets. The mechanisms of AS can be divided into 2 phases: The initiation phase is characterized by lipid-deposition, which generates inflammation in the valve leading to the propagation phase. The propagation phase is characterized by

an increased production of procalcific and pro-osteogenic factors in the valve leaflets, which leads to calcification of the valve and progression of AS.[10]

Calcific AS is also an adverse event associated with radiation therapy for cancer. With increased rates of survival after such therapy, radiation-induced AS has also largely increased. The aortic valve is not the only structure to calcify after thoracic radiation therapy, and it is most often associated with other calcifications on the mitral annulus, the aorta, the coronary arteries, and/or the pericardium.[11,12]

Association of HF and AS can be a matter of concomitance, such as concomitant AS and ischemic HF or amyloidosis, as there are shared risk factors and the possibility of amyloid infiltration of the valve leaflets,[13] or both caused by cancer treatment.[12] It can also be a cause and effect relationship, as HF is the evolution of untreated AS, because the increased afterload imposed by the stenotic valve leads to a decrease in the coronary flow reserve and cardiac hypertrophy—resulting in cardiac fibrosis and HF symptoms.[14,15]

Evaluation of Aortic Stenosis Severity by Rest Echocardiography

Regardless of the cause of HF symptoms, the first choice for assessing AS-severity is echocardiography.

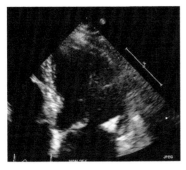

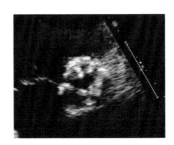

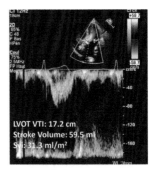

Aortic Valve – Short Axis View
Systole

Left Ventricle – End Diastole (up) and End Systole (down)

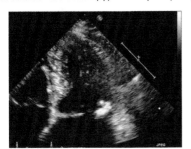

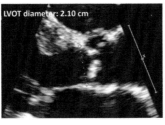

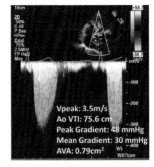

LV Outflow tract diameter

Fig. 2. Echocardiographic examination of a patient with aortic stenosis and preserved ejection fraction but with low flow. Ao, aorta; AVA, aortic valve area; LVOT, left ventricular outflow tract; SVi, stroke volume indexed to body surface area; Vpeak, peak aortic jet velocity; VTI, velocity-time integral.

Transthoracic Echocardiography

According to guidelines, the assessment of AS-severity is primarily based on the measurement of aortic peak velocity, aortic mean gradient and calculation of AVA.[16,17] Severe AS is described as a peak aortic velocity of 4.0 m/s or greater, aortic mean gradient of 40 mm Hg or greater, and AVA of less than 1.0 cm^2 (**Table 1**).

However, many patients with AS and concomitant HF present with discordant echocardiographic findings with a small AVA but lower than expected aortic mean gradient and aortic peak velocity.[18,19]

These findings could result from measurement errors, such as poor alignment of the Doppler flow or underestimation of the left ventricular outflow tract. Therefore, the first step when facing a discordant echocardiographic grading is to rule out any measurement errors.[3,4] If still discordant, assessing flow state is called for, especially in patients with preserved ejection fraction. Current guidelines agree, that a low flow state is present when stroke volume indexed to body surface area (SVi) is less than 35.0 mL/m^2, and if present with reduced ejection, fraction is called classic low-flow low-gradient AS or paradoxical low-flow low-gradient AS if ejection fraction is preserved.

However, SVi does not represent flow rate per se, which is calculated by dividing stroke volume

by LV ejection time.[16,17] Flow rate of less than 200 mL/s is considered low and has been found to be a prognostic marker in patients with AS and low flow, especially in patients with bradycardia.[20–22] However, flow rate is considered normal at 250 mL/s or greater, which unfortunately leaves a gray zone between 200 and 250 mL/s.

When flow is decreased, guidelines suggest evaluation of secondary echocardiographic measurements that could indicated AS-severity, such as indexed aortic valve area (AVAi) and velocity-ratio or VTI-ratio with AS being considered severe if AVAi is 0.6 cm^2/m^2 or less or with ratio of 0.25 or less.[23] However, both these parameters are also flow-dependent and not more accurate than AVA when low flow state is present. Thus, other imaging modalities must be used to ascertain the AS-severity.[3,4]

Transesophageal Echocardiography

Transesophageal echocardiography (TEE) is no longer routinely recommended in the assessment of patients with AS.[16] However, in patients with suboptimal transthoracic echocardiography (TTE) images, TEE may be helpful in improving image quality as well as provide insight into aortic valve anatomy. With TEE, planimetry of the aortic valve is possible but it is not considered a reliable method of determining AS-severity because it

Table 1
Criteria for aortic stenosis severity grading

	Aortic Stenosis Severity		
	Mild	Moderate	Severe
Rest Echocardiography			
Peak Aortic jet velocity (m/s)	2.6–3.0	3.0–4.0	>4.0
Mean gradient (mm Hg)	<25	25–40	>40
Aortic valve area (cm^2)	>1.5	1.5–1.0	<1.0
Doppler velocity index	>0.50	0.25–0.50	<0.25
Dobutamine Stress Echocardiography			
Stress mean gradient (mm Hg)			>40
Stress aortic valve area (cm^2)			<1.0
Projected AVA (cm^2)			<1.0
Computed tomography			
Aortic valve calcification (AU)			Women: >1200 Men: >2000
AVC density* (AU/cm^2)			Women: >300 Men: >500

* AVC density is the AVC divided by the sex-specific threshod identifying severe aortic stenosis (ie, 1200AU in women and 2000AU in men).

measures the geometric area of the valve and not the effective orifice area.[24] Indeed, the flow directed to converge at a narrow orifice will continue to converge beyond it, until interaction with the surrounding fluid cause divergence (**Fig. 3**). Thus, the effective orifice area is always smaller than the geometric one with an approximate ratio of 0.6 to 1 but low-flow rate can affect geometric valve area as well because the valve might not be fully opened by the flow.[24]

Diagnostic Approach in Discordant Echocardiographic Measurements

As resting echocardiography (TTE and TEE) is not able to ascertain AS-severity in case of discordant grading, it is mandatory to perform further examination in order to assess the actual AS-severity.

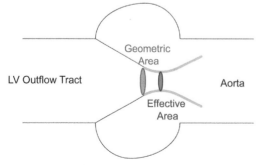

LV Outflow Tract — Geometric Area — Effective Area — Aorta

Fig. 3. Schema of geometric and effective aortic valve area.

Dobutamine Stress Echocardiography

In patients with reduced ejection fraction, guidelines recommend performing dobutamine stress echocardiography (DSE) to differentiate between true-severe and pseudosevere AS. A protocol of 5 μg/kg/min increments until a max dosage of 20μg/kg/min is recommended.[23] The criterions for true-severe AS is if peak velocity of 4.0 m/s or greater or aortic mean gradient of 40 mm Hg or greater with an AVA less than 1.0 cm^2 at any given time during DSE[16,23] (**Fig. 4**).

However, several patients will not reach a normal flow state during DSE, and because these parameters are all flow-dependent, DSE ends up being inconclusive with a continued low AVA but without concordant high peak velocity or mean gradient.

Projected aortic valve area
In patients with inconclusive DSE, the calculation of the projected AVA at a normal flow rate can help in the assessment of AS-severity.[25,26]

$$AVA_{proj} = AVA_{Rest} + \frac{AVA_{Peak} - AVA_{Rest}}{Q_{Peak} - Q_{Rest}}$$
$$\times (250 - Q_{Rest})$$

with Q being the flow rate and Rest and Peak being AVA or Q values at rest and at peak dobutamine stress.

A projected AVA of 1.0 cm^2 or lesser suggests the presence of true-severe AS (see **Fig. 4**) and

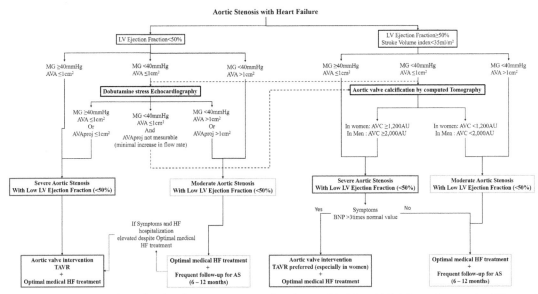

Fig. 4. Central Figure: Algorithm for the management of patients with AS and HF. AS, aortic stenosis; AVA, aortic valve area; AVAproj, projected aortic valve area; HF, heart failure; LV, left ventricular; MG, mean gradient; TAVR, transcatheter aortic valve replacement.

has been shown to be associated with increased mortality in patients with HFpEF.[27] However, in patients with HFrEF, a projected AVA of 1.2 cm² or lesser was associated with mortality,[25,28] meaning that pseudosevere AS may be detrimental in patients with HFrEF.

Of note, projected AVA cannot be calculated if the increase in flow rate is minimal (ie, <15%), due to the high variability of the projection line.

Cardiac-multidetector computer tomography
Cardiac-multidetector computer tomography (C-MDCT) allows for the measurement of calcification and can be used to quantify calcification in both coronaries and valves using the Agatston method (**Fig. 5**).[29,30] C-MDCT has been shown to be highly accurate for quantification of the aortic valve calcification (AVC) and has been shown to be correlated to the hemodynamic AS-severity.[31,32] Furthermore, AVC is a flow-independent measurement of AS-severity and has been shown to be highly reproducible.[33]

However, several studies have demonstrated that women reach a similar AS hemodynamic severity as men but with a lower AVC score. Thus, sex-specific thresholds for the definition of severe AS have been proposed; an AVC-score of 1200 (or 1300) AU or greater in woman and 2000 AU or greater in men indicates severe AS[31,34,35] (see **Fig. 4**). The sex-specific thresholds have been validated in many studies and add incremental value to predict AS progression and outcomes.[35–37]

AVC do have some limitation in its use, especially when the cause of AS is more associated with fibrosis than calcification, such as young patients with a bicuspid aortic valve or patients with amyloidosis.[38–40] In the setting of AS with HFpEF, amyloidosis is unfortunately not rare, and red flags should prompt the physician to confirm the diagnosis of amyloidosis.[13,41]

Evaluation of Myocardial Damage

Assessing myocardial damage as well as AS-severity is important. Myocardial damage impacts the outcome of AS treatment negatively, and low ejection fraction, low SVi as well as a low-flow state has all been shown to be associated with an increased mortality under medical management, and after both surgical and transcatheter aortic valve replacement (TAVR).[42–46]

Cardiac MRI

Cardiac MRI (C-MRI) is useful in both assessing extend of myocardial damage but also in characterizing both focal and diffuse fibrosis and is considered the gold standard for assessing myocardial damage.[47] Almost half of all patients with severe AS present with some degree of myocardial scar tissue, and the prevalence is even higher in patients with low SVi.[15,48]

Although focal fibrosis does not decrease after AVR, diffuse fibrosis could be reversible.[49,50] However, both focal and diffuse fibrosis have been

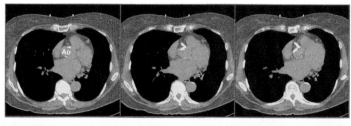
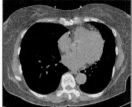
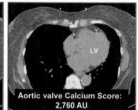
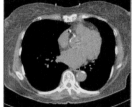
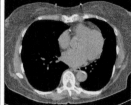

Multidetector Computed Tomography
- 120KV
- mAs according to patient body weight
- R-R interval: 60–80%
- Slice thickness: 3mm

Yellow (by software): >130Hounsfield Unit
Pink: selected by operator as aortic valve

Aortic valve Calcium Score: 2,760 AU

Fig. 5. Multidetector scan of a patient with severe aortic valve calcification. Ao, aorta; LV, left ventricle.

shown to be associated with a worse prognosis in AS, both in patients under medical treatment or undergoing AVR.[51–53] Accordingly early AVR in asymptomatic patients based on C-MRI could be beneficial in some patients with AS (especially those with HF).[54] This hypothesis is currently being tested in an ongoing study (NCT03094143).

However, C-MRI do have some limitations, it is time-consuming and may not always be available or feasible. As such, several biomarkers have been tested as surrogate markers for myocardial fibrosis in risk stratification in patients with AS and to guide therapeutic decision-making.

Global Longitudinal Strain

Reduction in ejection fraction is a late marker of LV dysfunction in AS, and a marker of "subclinical" LV dysfunction could be beneficial. Many studies have demonstrated that longitudinal strain is a sensitive marker to detect subclinical myocardial impairment when LVEF is preserved and can be used as a marker for risk stratification in patients with AS and reduced ejection fraction.[55–60]

Brain Natriuretic Peptide and N-terminal proBNP

Brain natriuretic peptide (BNP) and N-terminal proBNP (NT-proBNP) are peptides secreted by the LV in response to mechanic stress cause by an increase pressure or volume. Several studies have demonstrated a link between BNP or NT-proBNP and outcomes in AS.[61–64] However, the threshold to identify patient at risk have been highly variable from one study to the other. This is most likely related to the fact that both BNP and NTpro-BNP increases with age and normal reference has

been shown to be higher in women.[65] Furthermore, measurements of both BNP and NT-proBNP are highly dependent on the assay used, especially BNP.

This problem has been accommodated with BNP-ratio, that is, measured BNP divided by the highest normal value expected for the age and sex of the patient and the assay used.[66] BNP-ratio has been shown to independently predict mortality in both symptomatic and asymptomatic patients with AS and preserved ejection fraction.[66] In patients with decreased ejection fraction, NT-proBNP seems to have superior prognostic value than BNP.[67]

High-Sensitivity Troponin (I and T)

Plasma high-sensitivity troponin is well documented in term of both diagnostic and prognostic value in patients with coronary artery disease. In patients with AS, high-sensitivity troponin has been shown to be associated with a higher fibrosis and hypertrophy burden and an increased mortality.[68,69] In addition, high-sensitivity troponin could be associated to BNP or NT-proBNP and/or other biomarkers to refine risk stratification in AS.[70] However, troponins are not proposed in the current guidelines for the risk stratification in AS.

Management of Patient with Aortic Stenosis

AS is a progressive disease. Progression rate is highly variable from one patient to the other and is influenced by several genetic and environmental risk factors such as age, lipoprotein (a), Low-Density-Lipoprotein cholesterol, hypertension, and so forth,[71,72] as well as the severity of the stenosis. Indeed, the level of calcification in the valve and the hemodynamic severity of AS are the most powerful predictor of rapid progression. The median (95% confidence interval) rate of progression of AS is an increase of 4.1 (2.80–5.41) mm Hg/y of mean gradient, 0.19 (0.13–0.24) m/s/y of peak aortic jet velocity, 158.5 (55.0–261.9) AU/y of AVC, and a decrease of −0.08 (0.06–0.10) cm²/y of AVA,[73] with the fastest rate of progression for the most severe AS.

Medical Treatment in Patients with Heart Failure and Aortic Stenosis

No medical treatment has yet been shown to influence the progression of AS. However, optimal medical therapy for HF is essential and should be optimized in order to reduce the afterload burden. Guideline-directed medical therapy is characterized by addressing risk factors with both nonpharmacological and pharmacological treatment of HF, hypertension, and dyslipidemia.

Aortic Valve Replacement in Patients with Severe Aortic Stenosis

Guidelines recommend AVR if AS is severe with high gradient, and patient is either symptomatic or has reduced ejection fraction (class I).[16,17] For symptomatic patients with discordant echocardiographic findings and low SVi, AVR is recommended (Class I) if AS is determined to be true severe by further examination and AS is determined to be the most likely cause of symptoms.[16,17]

For asymptomatic patients with preserved ejection fraction and severe AS, AVR is recommended if the patient demonstrates symptoms during exercise testing (Class I) or with an abnormal exercise testing (drop in blood pressure - Class IIa), or if AS is very severe with peak aortic velocity of greater than 5.0 m/s or aortic mean gradient greater than 60 mm Hg, if AS is progressing rapidly (peak aortic velocity progression ≥0.3 m/s/y), or BNP is markedly elevated (>3 times the normal age-corrected and sex-corrected value), or if LVEF <60% on at least 3 serial imaging studies.[16,17]

Choice of Intervention

The choice of intervention, that is, SAVR or TAVR is a shared decision-making with a well-informed patient and depends on aorta and aortic valve anatomy, age (or life expectancy), comorbidity, and surgical risk (STS-PROM/EuroSCORE II). In patients aged younger than 50 years, SAVR with mechanical aortic valve prosthesis is recommended, unless the patient has a contraindication to anticoagulation treatment.

In older patients, recommendation differs between guidelines. As a general rule, the recommendation for patients aged 70 years or younger, long life expectancy and with a low surgical risk (STS-PROM/EuroSCORE II <4%) is SAVR, and the recommendation for patients aged 75 years or older, short life expectancy or with a high surgical risk (STS-PROM/EuroSCORE II >8%) is TAVR.[16,17]

One should remember that patients with low ejection fraction are at high surgical risk, and that patients with low SVi have a higher surgical risk than calculated by current risk score.[44,46] Furthermore, SAVR carries an inherent risk of prosthesis-patient mismatch, especially in women with a small aortic-annulus[74] (see **Fig. 4**).

In some cases, balloon aortic valvuloplasty may be considered as palliative treatment or as a bridge to AVR in patients where AVR is unfeasible. Balloon aortic valvuloplasty carries its own risk of complications and has not been demonstrated to decrease either mortality or morbidity in patients with AS but does decrease the HF hospitalization burden.[75,76]

Aortic Valve Replacement in Patients with Moderate Aortic Stenosis

AVR could only be considered in patients with moderate AS if another open-heart surgery is planned (class IIb).[16,17] However, recent studies have suggested that patient with moderate AS and LVEF of less than 50% have a worse prognosis then expected, with a higher burden of HF hospitalization and increased mortality.[7,77] In these patients, AVR and especially transfemoral TAVR could improve the survival (see **Fig. 4**). Randomized control trials are ongoing to examine the clinical benefit of AVR in patients with moderate AS and HF: the "Transcatheter Aortic Valve Replacement to UNload the Left ventricle in patients with ADvanced heart failure" (TAVR UNLOAD) trial and the "Management of Moderate Aortic Stenosis by Clinical Surveillance or TAVR" (PROGRESS) trial.[78]

Furthermore, a number of large randomized control trials examining the timing of intervention in asymptomatic patients with severe or moderate-severe AS are expected in the near-future (NCT03042104 and NCT03972644).

SUMMARY

The decision of intervention in AS patients with HF depends almost exclusively on AS-severity but in patients with HF, echocardiographic evaluation of AS-severity can be inconclusive due to discordant measurements, and further examination is required. When AS is determined to be severe, the choice of intervention (SAVR or TAVR) can be difficult given that patients with HF often are at intermediate-to-high operative risk, even with preserved ejection fraction. Nevertheless, the decision regarding the type of intervention should be discussed with the patient, and based on age, surgical risk, life expectancy, and preference of the patient. Finally, patients with HFrEF and moderate AS might benefit from intervention; however, there is no recommendation for AVR in the current guideline (except if concomitant open-heart surgery is planned). Ongoing studies are examining the clinical significance of AVR in patients with moderate AS and HF as well as the timing of AVR in asymptomatic patients with severe or moderate-severe AS.

CLINICS CARE POINTS

- Medical treatment for HF should be optimized concurrently with the determination of AS severity.
- Measurement errors should be ruled out in patients with discordant echocardiographic findings, and if discordance is confirmed, additional imaging modality must be used.
- The choice of intervention should be shared decision-making, reminding that patients with HF are at high/higher surgical risk.

DISCLOSURES

Dr Clavel received funding from Edwards Lifesciences (United States) for computed tomography core laboratory analyses in the field of surgical aortic valve prosthesis with no direct personal compensation and research grant from Medtronic (United States). The other authors have no conflict of interest relevant to the contents of this article to declare.

REFERENCES

1. Lindman BR, Clavel MA, Mathieu P, et al. Calcific aortic stenosis. Nat Rev Dis Primers 2016;2:16006.
2. Frank S, Johnson A, Ross JJ Jr. Natural history of valvular aortic stenosis. Br Heart J 1973;35:41–6.
3. Clavel MA, Magne J, Pibarot P. Low-gradient aortic stenosis. Eur Heart J 2016;37(34):2645–57.
4. Clavel MA, Burwash IG, Pibarot P. Cardiac imaging for assessing low-gradient severe aortic stenosis. JACC Cardiovasc Imaging 2017;10(2):185–202.
5. Smith CR, Leon MB, Mack MJ, et al. Transcatheter versus surgical aortic-valve replacement in high-risk patients. N Engl J Med 2011;364(23):2187–98.
6. Guzzetti E, Annabi MS, Pibarot P, et al. Multimodality imaging for discordant low-gradient aortic stenosis: assessing the valve and the myocardium. Frontiers in Cardiovascular Medicine: Cardiovascular Imaging 2020;7:570689.
7. Jean G, Van Mieghem NM, Gegenava T, et al. Moderate aortic stenosis in patients with heart failure and reduced ejection fraction. J Am Coll Cardiol 2021;77(22):2796–803.
8. Roberts WC. The structure of the aortic valve in clinically isolated aortic stenosis. An autopsy study of 162 patients over 15 years of age. Circulation 1970;XLII(7):91–7.
9. Eveborn GW, Schirmer H, Heggelund G, et al. The evolving epidemiology of valvular aortic stenosis. The Tromso Study. Heart 2013;99(6):396–400.
10. Pawade TA, Newby DE, Dweck MR. Calcification in aortic stenosis: The skeleton key. J Am Coll Cardiol 2015;66(5):561–77.
11. Mitchell JD, Cehic DA, Morgia M, et al. Cardiovascular Manifestations From Therapeutic Radiation: A Multidisciplinary Expert Consensus Statement From the International Cardio-Oncology Society. JACC CardioOncology 2021;3(3):360–80.
12. Belzile-Dugas E, Fremes S, Eisenberg MJ. Radiation-Induced Aortic Stenosis: An Update on Treatment Modalities. JACC (J Am Coll Cardiol): Advances 2023;2(1):1–10.
13. Ternacle J, Krapf L, Mohty D, et al. Aortic stenosis and cardiac amyloidosis: JACC review topic of the week. J Am Coll Cardiol 2019;74(21):2638–51.
14. Hein S, Arnon E, Kostin S, et al. Progression from compensated hypertrophy to failure in the pressure-overloaded human heart: structural deterioration and compensatory mechanisms. Circulation 2003;107(7):984–91.
15. Weidemann F, Herrmann S, Stork S, et al. Impact of myocardial fibrosis in patients with symptomatic severe aortic stenosis. Circulation 2009;120(7):577–84.
16. Otto CM, Nishimura RA, Bonow RO, et al. 2020 ACC/AHA guideline for the management of patients with valvular heart disease: executive summary: A report of the American College of Cardiology/American Heart Association joint committee on clinical practice guidelines. J Am Coll Cardiol 2021;77(4):450–500.
17. Vahanian A, Beyersdorf F, Praz F, et al. 2021 ESC/EACTS guidelines for the management of valvular heart disease. Eur Heart J 2022;43:561–632.
18. Connolly HM, Oh JK, Schaff HV, et al. Severe aortic stenosis with low transvalvular gradient and severe left ventricular dysfunction. Result of aortic valve replacement in 52 patients. Circulation 2000;101:1940–6.
19. Clavel MA, Pibarot P, Dumesnil JG. Paradoxical low flow aortic valve stenosis: incidence, evaluation,

and clinical significance. Curr Cardiol Rep 2014; 16(1):431.

20. Vamvakidou A, Jin W, Danylenko O, et al. Impact of pre-intervention transaortic flow rate versus stroke volume index on mortality across the hemodynamic spectrum of severe aortic stenosis: implications for a new hemodynamic classification of aortic stenosis. JACC Cardiovasc Imaging 2019;12(1):205–6.

21. Sen J, Huynh Q, Stub D, et al. Prognosis of severe low-flow, low-gradient aortic stenosis by stroke volume index and transvalvular flow rate. JACC Cardiovasc Imaging 2021;14(5):915–27.

22. Clavel MA, Annabi MS. Low-flow aortic stenosis: flow rate does not replace but could refine stroke volume index. JACC Cardiovasc Imaging 2021; 14(5):928–30.

23. Baumgartner H, Hung J, Bermejo J, et al. Recommendations on the echocardiographic assessment of aortic valve stenosis: A focused update from the European Association of Cardiovascular Imaging and the American Society of Echocardiography. J Am Soc Echocardiogr 2017;30(4):372–92.

24. Gilon D, Cape EG, Handschumacher MD, et al. Effect of three-dimensional valve shape on the hemodynamics of aortic stenosis: three-dimensional echocardiograpic stereolithography and patient studies. J Am Coll Cardiol 2002;40:1479–86.

25. Clavel MA, Burwash IG, Mundigler G, et al. Validation of conventional and simplified methods to calculate projected valve area at normal flow rate in patients with low flow, low gradient aortic stenosis: the multicenter TOPAS (True or Pseudo Severe Aortic Stenosis) study. J Am Soc Echocardiogr 2010;23(4):380–6.

26. Blais C, Burwash IG, Mundigler G, et al. Projected valve area at normal flow rate improves the assessment of stenosis severity in patients with low flow, low-gradient aortic stenosis: The multicenter TOPAS (Truly or Pseudo Severe Aortic Stenosis) study. Circulation 2006;113(5):711–21.

27. Clavel MA, Ennezat PV, Marechaux S, et al. Stress echocardiography to assess stenosis severity and predict outcome in patients with paradoxical low-flow, low-gradient aortic stenosis and preserved LVEF. J Am Coll Cardiol Img 2013;6(2):175–83.

28. Clavel MA, Fuchs C, Burwash IG, et al. Predictors of outcomes in low-flow, low-gradient aortic stenosis: results of the multicenter TOPAS Study. Circulation 2008;118(14 Suppl):S234–42.

29. Agatston AS, Janowitz WR, Hildner FJ, et al. Quantification of coronary artery calcium using ultrafast computed tomography. J Am Coll Cardiol 1990; 15(4):827–32.

30. Pawade T, Sheth T, Guzzetti E, et al. Why and how to measure aortic valve calcification in patients with aortic stenosis. JACC Cardiovasc Imaging 2019; 12(9):1835–48.

31. Aggarwal SR, Clavel MA, Messika-Zeitoun D, et al. Sex differences in aortic valve calcification measured by multidetector computed tomography in aortic stenosis. Circ Cardiovasc Imaging 2013;6(1):40–7.

32. Linde L, Carter-Storch R, Christensen NL, et al. Sex differences in aortic valve calcification in severe aortic valve stenosis: association between computer tomography assessed calcification and valvular calcium concentrations. Eur Heart J Cardiovasc Imaging 2021;22:581–8.

33. Doris MK, Jenkins W, Robson P, et al. Computed tomography aortic valve calcium scoring for the assessment of aortic stenosis progression. Heart 2020;106(24):1906–13.

34. Clavel MA, Messika-Zeitoun D, Pibarot P, et al. The complex nature of discordant severe calcified aortic valve disease grading: New insights from combined Doppler-echocardiographic and computed tomographic study. J Am Coll Cardiol 2013;62(24):2329–38.

35. Pawade T, Clavel MA, Tribouilloy C, et al. Computed tomography aortic valve calcium scoring in patients with aortic stenosis. Circ Cardiovasc Imaging 2018; 11(3):e007146.

36. Clavel MA, Pibarot P, Messika-Zeitoun D, et al. Impact of aortic valve calcification, as measured by MDCT, on survival in patients with aortic stenosis: results of an international registry study. J Am Coll Cardiol 2014;64(12):1202–13.

37. Tastet L, Enriquez-Sarano M, Capoulade R, et al. Impact of aortic valve calcification and sex on hemodynamic progression and clinical outcomes in AS. J Am Coll Cardiol 2017;69(16):2096–8.

38. Shen M, Tastet L, Capoulade R, et al. Effect of age and aortic valve anatomy on calcification and haemodynamic severity of aortic stenosis. Heart 2017; 103(1):32–9.

39. Voisine M, Hervault M, Shen M, et al. Age, sex, and valve phenotype differences in fibro-calcific remodeling of calcified aortic valve. J Am Heart Assoc 2020;e015610.

40. Hussain M, Hanna M, Griffin BP, et al. Aortic valve calcium in patients with transthyretin cardiac amyloidosis: A propensity-matched analysis. Circ Cardiovasc Imaging 2020;13(10):e011433.

41. Cavalcante JL, Rijal S, Abdelkarim I, et al. Cardiac amyloidosis is prevalent in older patients with aortic stenosis and carries worse prognosis. J Cardiovasc Magn Reson 2017;19(1):98.

42. Monin JL, Monchi M, Gest V, et al. Aortic stenosis with severe left ventricular dysfunction and low transvalvular pressure gradients. J Am Coll Cardiol 2001;37(8):2101–7.

43. Hachicha Z, Dumesnil JG, Bogaty P, et al. Paradoxical low flow, low gradient severe aortic stenosis despite preserved ejection fraction is associated with higher afterload and reduced survival. Circulation 2007;115(22):2856–64.

44. Le Ven F, Freeman M, Webb J, et al. Impact of low flow on the outcome of high risk patients undergoing transcatheter aortic valve replacement. J Am Coll Cardiol 2013;62(9):782–8.

45. Clavel MA, Berthelot-Richer M, LV F, et al. Impact of classic and paradoxical low flow on survival after aortic valve replacement for severe aortic stenosis. J Am Coll Cardiol 2015;65(7):645–53.

46. Guzzetti E, Poulin A, Annabi MS, et al. Transvalvular flow, sex, and survival after valve replacement surgery in patients with severe aortic stenosis. J Am Coll Cardiol 2020;75(16):1897–909.

47. Salerno M, Sharif B, Arheden H, et al. Recent Advances in Cardiovascular Magnetic Resonance: Techniques and Applications. Circ Cardiovasc Imaging 2017;10(6).

48. Musa TA, Treibel TA, Vassiliou VS, et al. Myocardial scar and mortality in severe aortic stenosis. Circulation 2018;138(18):1935–47.

49. Arbustini E, Weidemann F, Hall JL. Reply: The importance of cardiac cycle in the imaging criteria for left ventricular noncompaction. J Am Coll Cardiol 2015; 65(13):1383–4.

50. Everett RJ, Tastet L, Clavel MA, et al. Progression of hypertrophy and myocardial fibrosis in aortic stenosis: A multicenter cardiac magnetic resonance study. Circ Cardiovasc Imaging 2018;11(6):e007451.

51. Everett RJ, Treibel TA, Fukui M, et al. Extracellular myocardial volume in patients with aortic stenosis. J Am Coll Cardiol 2020;75(3):304–16.

52. Chin CW, Everett RJ, Kwiecinski J, et al. Myocardial fibrosis and cardiac decompensation in aortic stenosis. JACC Cardiovasc Imaging 2017;10(11):1320–33.

53. Herrmann S, Stork S, Niemann M, et al. Low-gradient aortic valve stenosis: Myocardial fibrosis and its influence on function and outcome. J Am Coll Cardiol 2011;58(4):402–12.

54. Chin CW, Messika-Zeitoun D, Shah AS, et al. A clinical risk score of myocardial fibrosis predicts adverse outcomes in aortic stenosis. Eur Heart J 2016;37(8):713–23.

55. Carstensen HG, Larsen LH, Hassager C, et al. Basal longitudinal strain predicts future aortic valve replacement in asymptomatic patients with aortic stenosis. Eur Heart J Cardiovasc Imaging 2016; 17(3):283–92.

56. Pibarot P, Dumesnil JG. Longitudinal myocardial shortening in aortic stenosis: Ready for prime time after 30 years of research? Heart 2009;96(2):95–6.

57. Donal E, Thebault C, O'Connor K, et al. Impact of aortic stenosis on longitudinal myocardial deformation during exercise. Eur J Echocardiogr 2011; 12(3):235–41.

58. Dahou A, Bartko PE, Capoulade R, et al. Usefulness of global left ventricular longitudinal strain for risk stratification in low ejection fraction, low-gradient aortic stenosis: results from the multicenter True or Pseudo-Severe Aortic Stenosis study. Circ Cardiovasc Imaging 2015;8(3):e002117.

59. Magne J, Cosyns B, Popescu BA, et al. Distribution and prognostic significance of left ventricular global longitudinal strain in asymptomatic significant aortic stenosis: An individual participant data meta-analysis. JACC Cardiovasc Imaging 2019;12(1):84–92.

60. Huded CP, Masri A, Kusunose K, et al. Outcomes in asymptomatic severe aortic stenosis with preserved ejection fraction undergoing rest and treadmill stress echocardiography. J Am Heart Assoc 2018; 7(8).

61. Bergler-Klein J, Klaar U, Heger M, et al. Natriuretic Peptides Predict Symptom-Free Survival and Post-operative Outcome in Severe Aortic Stenosis. Circulation 2004;109:2302–8.

62. Chen S, Redfors B, O'Neill BP, et al. Low and elevated B-type natriuretic peptide levels are associated with increased mortality in patients with preserved ejection fraction undergoing transcatheter aortic valve replacement: an analysis of the PARTNER II trial and registry. Eur Heart J 2020;41(8):958–69.

63. Nguyen V, Cimadevilla C, Arangalage D, et al. Determinants and prognostic value of B-type natriuretic peptide in patients with aortic valve stenosis. Int J Cardiol 2017;230:371–7.

64. Nessmith MG, Brucks S, Little WC. Elevated B-type natriuretic peptide indicates poor survival in aortic stenosis. Circulation 2004;110(17). III–710.

65. Redfield M, Rodeheffer R, Jacobsen S, et al. Plasma brain natriuretic peptide concentration: impact of age and gender. J Am Coll Cardiol 2002;40(5): 976–82.

66. Clavel MA, Malouf J, Michelena HI, et al. B-type natriuretic peptide clinical activation in aortic stenosis: Impact on long-term survival. J Am Coll Cardiol 2014;63(19):2016–25.

67. Annabi MS, Zhang B, Bergler-Klein J, et al. Usefulness of the B-type natriuretic peptides in low ejection fraction, low flow, low-gradient aortic stenosis results from the TOPAS multicenter prospective cohort study. Structural Heart 2021;5(3):319–27.

68. Chin CW, Shah AS, McAllister DA, et al. High-sensitivity troponin I concentrations are a marker of an advanced hypertrophic response and adverse outcomes in patients with aortic stenosis. Eur Heart J 2014;35(34):2312–21.

69. Rosjo H, Andreassen J, Edvardsen T, et al. Prognostic usefulness of circulating high-sensitivity troponin T in aortic stenosis and relation to echocardiographic indexes of cardiac function and anatomy. Am J Cardiol 2011;108(1):88–91.

70. Dahou A, Clavel MA, Capoulade R, et al. B-Type natriuretic peptide and high-sensitivity cardiac troponin for risk stratification in low-flow, low-gradient aortic stenosis. JACC Cardiovasc Imaging 2018;11(7):939–47.

71. Tastet L, Capoulade R, Clavel MA, et al. Systolic hypertension and progression of aortic valve calcification in patients with aortic stenosis: results from the PROGRESSA study. Eur Heart J Cardiovasc Imaging 2017;18(1):70–8.

72. Capoulade R, Chan KL, Yeang C, et al. Oxidized phospholipids, lipoprotein(a), and progression of calcific aortic valve stenosis. J Am Coll Cardiol 2015;66(11):1236–46.

73. Willner N, Prosperi-Porta G, Lau L, et al. Aortic stenosis progression: a systematic review and meta-analysis, 2022. JACC Cardiovasc Imaging 2023; 16(3):314–28.

74. Cote N, Clavel MA. Sex differences in the pathophysiology, diagnosis, and management of aortic stenosis. Cardiol Clin 2020;38(1):129–38.

75. Mantovani F, Clavel MA, Potenza A, et al. Balloon aortic valvuloplasty as a palliative treatment in patients with severe aortic stenosis and limited life expectancy: a single center experience. Aging 2020;12(16):16597–608.

76. Szerlip M, Arsalan M, Mack MC, et al. Usefulness of Balloon Aortic Valvuloplasty in the Management of Patients With Aortic Stenosis. Am J Cardiol 2017; 120(8):1366–72.

77. van Gils L, Clavel MA, Vollema EM, et al. Prognostic implications of moderate aortic stenosis in patients with left ventricular systolic dysfunction. J Am Coll Cardiol 2017;69(19):2383–92.

78. Spitzer E, Van Mieghem NM, Pibarot P, et al. Rationale and design of the Transcatheter Aortic Valve Replacement to UNload the Left ventricle in patients with ADvanced heart failure (TAVR UNLOAD) trial. Am Heart J 2016;182:80–8.

Aortic Regurgitation and Heart Failure

Advances in Diagnosis, Management, and Interventions

Graham Peigh, MD, MSc*, Jyothy J. Puthumana, MD,
Robert O. Bonow, MD, MS

KEYWORDS

- Heart failure • Aortic regurgitation • Cardiovascular imaging

KEY POINTS

- Comorbid aortic regurgitation and heart failure exists on the spectrum of aortic regurgitation severity.
- While 2D transthoracic echocardiography is the primary technique to evaluate aortic regurgitation, 3D transthoracic echocardiography, cardiac magnetic resonance imaging and speckle tracking echocardiography may provide important prognostic data in specific populations.
- The only effective treatment of patients with symptomatic aortic regurgitation or those with severe left ventricular dilation or reduced left ventricular ejection fraction at risk for heart failure, is operative management.
- Select patients who necessitate operative management of aortic regurgitation, but are not candidates for surgical aortic valve replacement, may benefit from off-label transcatheter-based therapies.

INTRODUCTION

Aortic regurgitation (AR), characterized by diastolic flow reversal through the aortic valve (AV), is a common valvular abnormality with a prevalence of 5% to 13% in population-based studies.[1] AR may occur due to a primary defect in AV structure/function, or in a secondary fashion due to abnormalities in the proximal ascending aorta.[2] In developing countries, rheumatic heart disease is the leading etiology of AR. Conversely, in developed countries, bicuspid AV disease, degenerated AV leaflets, or annuloaortic ectasia are the most common causes of AR. [2,3]

Recent guidelines isolate four progressive stages of AR based on clinical risk factors, valve anatomy, valve function, myocardial function, and patient symptoms. The stages range from those at risk for developing AR based on risk factors (Grade A) to those with severe symptomatic AR and heart failure (HF) symptoms (Grade D).[3]

Patients with mild AR may be asymptomatic or even have increased exercise capacity,[4] and the natural time course of AR progression is oftentimes slow. However, when AR does progress, the augmented regurgitant volume into the left ventricle (LV) causes increased LV preload and afterload, and subsequent LV remodeling via interstitial fibrosis and eccentric LV hypertrophy and dilation.[3] As the LV remodels, a cycle ensues which leads to additional interstitial fibrosis, decreased LV compliance, increased end-systolic volume/end-diastolic pressure, subsequent further LV dilation, and progressively increased volumes of regurgitant flow. Functionally, these changes can ultimately lead to decreased left ventricular ejection fraction (LVEF),

Division of Cardiology, Northwestern University, Feinberg School of Medicine, 676 North St. Clair Suite 600, Chicago, IL 60611, USA
* Corresponding author. Northwestern Memorial Hospital.
E-mail address: graham.peigh@northwestern.edu

Heart Failure Clin 19 (2023) 285–296
https://doi.org/10.1016/j.hfc.2023.02.007

heartfailure.theclinics.com

increased pressures throughout the cardiovascular system, and clinical HF.[5]

Comorbid AR and HF (AR-HF) is an entity on the spectrum of AR severity. This review discusses contemporary strategies in diagnosis, management, and intervention of AR-HF. Because HF is on the continuum of AR severity, this review will also discuss diagnostic techniques for pure AR, to further stratify who should be followed closely for incident clinical HF (**Fig. 1**).

EVALUATION

In this section, we will review the range of imaging, procedural and laboratory tests that may be used to evaluate AR-HF. Although a suggestive physical exam, laboratory testing, and transthoracic echocardiography (TTE) are the pillars of AR evaluation, utilization of speckle tracking echocardiography,

3-dimensional (3D) echocardiography, and cardiac magnetic resonance have provided significant advances in AR-HF evaluation (**Table 1**).

Physical Examination

The cardiovascular physical exam has historically been a mainstay in AR diagnosis. Numerous physical examination findings including a water hammer (Corrigan) pulse, de Musset's sign, and Muller sign may raise suspicion for AR. In addition, AR is characterized by a blowing diastolic decrescendo murmur that may extend for the duration of diastole.[6,7] There is often a systolic outflow murmur as well, related to the increased forward stroke volume, and it is not uncommon for the systolic murmur to be more obvious than the diastolic murmur.

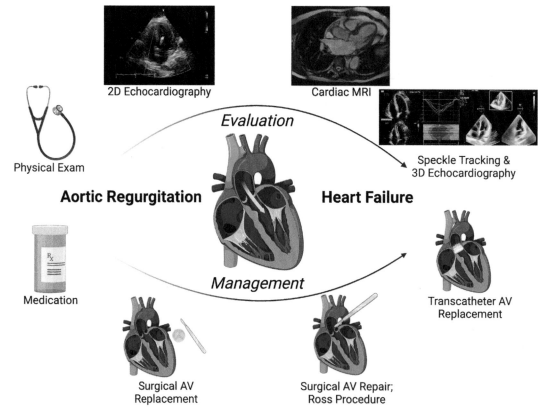

Fig. 1. Evaluation and management of AR and HF. Evaluation of AR and HF ranges from a comprehensive physical examination to imaging modalities including 2D echocardiography and cardiac MRI. In certain clinical situations, there are benefits to speckle tracking and 3D echocardiography, however, specific thresholds to define severe AR have not been defined using these imaging modalities. Not pictured are transesophageal echocardiography, laboratory assessment, and invasive angiography, all of which have unique clinical applicability. All patients with AR should have hypertension treated to target systolic blood pressure less than 140 mm Hg. The mainstay of management for AR and HF is surgical AVR. Specific patients, particularly those who are young, may benefit more from surgical AV repair or the Ross procedure. Data are forthcoming about the safety and efficacy of TAVR in cohorts with AR. 2D, 2-dimensional; 3D, 3-dimensional; AV, aortic valve; MRI, magnetic resonance imaging. (Created with BioRender.com)

Table 1
Imaging modalities to evaluate aortic regurgitation and heart failure

Method	Advantages	Disadvantages
2D transthoracic echocardiography	• Widely available and guideline recommended • Significant data on parameters associated with AR severity • Ability to simultaneously assess AV apparatus and LV structure/function • Can assess diastolic flow reversal in descending aorta	• Variability in image acquisition between users • Potential for foreshortening leading to underestimation of AR severity, LV ejection fraction, and LV volume • Difficult to calculate effective regurgitant orifice area or regurgitant volume
3D transthoracic echocardiography	• Superior ability to capture eccentric jets of AF • Comprehensive visualization of AV apparatus • Valid LVEF measurements	• Variability in image acquisition between users • Technology not widely available • Specific thresholds for severity of AR not yet defined
Speckle tracking echocardiography	• Cost-effective technique to detect subtle changes in myocardial dynamics • Technology readily available • Potential to post-process images if strain is not obtained on acquired images • Significant prognostic value in AR-HF	• Potential for inaccurate measurements due to LV foreshortening • Variability in image acquisition between users • Discrepant measurements between manufacturers • Does not assess for AR in isolation
Cardiac MRI	• Guideline recommended, particularly in patients with concomitant aortopathy or bicuspid AV • Superior ability to visualize eccentric jets of AR • Noninvasive method of evaluating LV fibrosis • Accurate measurement of LVEF • Incorporates interrogation of ascending aorta • May provide additional information about myocardial structure that predisposes to HF • Significant prognostic value in AR-HF	• Limited availability and increased cost • Requires patient participation • Claustrophobic patients may not be able to tolerate image acquisition • Unable to perform if patient has irregular R-R intervals
Transesophageal echocardiography	• Enhanced ability to visualize eccentric jets of AR • Circumferential view of AV to determine etiology of regurgitation • Ability to visualize descending aorta to evaluate for flow reversal • Provides prognostic information about ability for AV to be repaired, rather than replaced, at time of surgery	• Invasive procedure • Suboptimal assessment of LV function
Cardiac catheterization	• May evaluate for degree of AR when other tests produce discrepant results or are unavailable	• Invasive procedure • Use of contrast is prohibitive in patients with comorbid renal disease

Abbreviations: AR, aortic regurgitation; AV, aortic valve; HF, heart failure; LV, left ventricle; LVEF, left ventricular ejection fraction.

Although these physical exam signs have various degrees of sensitivity and specificity for AR diagnosis, in light of the relative prevalence and decreasing cost of TTE, auscultatory findings are now routinely confirmed with echocardiography. Furthermore, TTE has increased sensitivity for detection of subtle AV disease when compared to auscultation alone. Indeed, among 142 patients with cardiac structural abnormalities, limited hand-held echocardiography demonstrated higher sensitivity for the detection of valve disease than isolated auscultation.[8]

Transthoracic Echocardiography

2-Dimensional echocardiography

Full Doppler echocardiography may comprehensively evaluate AR and presence of LV dysfunction through an integrative approach to cardiac structure and function.[9,10] Specific parameters assessed on TTE to determine the presence of AR include pressure half time of the regurgitant jet (which is more important in acute, compared with chronic, AR), color Doppler regurgitant jet size, vena contracta size, proximal isovelocity surface area radius, and the presence or absence of holodiastolic flow reversal in the descending aorta.[9] In addition, the effective regurgitant orifice area and regurgitant volume may be calculated using standard measurements obtained from a 2-dimensional (2D) TTE to provide further information about AR severity. As AR progresses, TTE is also useful in determining whether the LV has remodeled via eccentric dilation as a response to volume overload. Determining the degree of LV dilation and/or dysfunction is most important in risk stratification of those patients who may be at the highest risk for the development of clinical HF.

Limitations of 2-dimensional transthoracic echocardiography Due to its widespread applicability, major guideline committees propose TTE-based grading systems for AR severity.[3,10] However, TTE evaluation of AR is subject to error due to differences in acquisition technique, and user variability. In addition, calculated TTE measurements may be significantly impacted by image quality, eccentric jets outside the plane of view, and abnormal flow convergence shapes.[9] Specifically, it is sometimes difficult to calculate an effective regurgitant orifice area using TTE due to the oftentimes small regurgitant orifice area and the oblique nature of the regurgitant jet that may be underappreciated on 2D imaging. Furthermore, due to the elliptical nature of the LV outflow tract (LVOT) and mitral valve annulus, calculating regurgitant volume is also subject to error.[10] Accordingly, the American Society of Echocardiography recommends using LV end-diastolic volume index (LVEDVi), which is not subject to as much acquisition error as functional parameters, as the primary echocardiographic parameter to grade AR severity. LV end-systolic volume index (LVESVi) and LVEF (derived from the LV volume data) also are important measures of LV dilation and systolic function.[11] Other calculated measures such as vena contracta, effective regurgitant orifice area regurgitant jet width, and holodiastolic flow reversal are to be used as secondary parameters.[10]

Advances to 2-Dimensional Echocardiography

3-Dimensional echocardiography

In addition to 2D acquisition techniques, contemporary TTE acquisition can include 3D reconstruction of various cardiac structures. Recently, 3D TTE has gained popularity in the evaluation of AR due to its ability to interrogate the AV without many of the limitations inherent to 2D imaging.[12] Whereas 2D TTE is subject to error due to oblique sectional planes, 3D reconstruction allows for holistic views of the AV apparatus.[12] Specific advantages of 3D TTE include superior characterization of the mechanisms for AR and greater accuracy in determining LVOT and aortic dimensions, and the effective regurgitant orifice area.[12] In addition, functional parameters including vena contracta measurement are enhanced by 3D TTE.[13] Particularly in patients with eccentric jets, 3D TTE confers significant advantage over 2D TTE in estimating regurgitant volume.[13] In addition, 3D TTE accurately measures LVEF, with results rivaling that of 2D TTE.[14] Taken together, the use of 3D TTE by experienced sonographers may be superior to that of 2D TTE in comprehensively evaluating AR and detecting the subset of patients who have severe LV dilation and/or LV systolic dysfunction and may thus be prone to developing clinical HF.

Speckle tracking echocardiography

Speckle tracking echocardiography, or strain imaging, provides information about myocardial dynamics by following, and quantifying, displacement of individual speckles across the cardiac cycle.[15] As such, strain imaging of the LV (global longitudinal strain) can quantify subtle changes in myocardial dynamics that are associated with eventual LV dilation or reduction in LVEF, before development of structural or functional abnormalities.[16–21] In addition, multiple studies have demonstrated the prognostic ability of global longitudinal strain in patients with severe AR.[16–20] Indeed, among a cohort of patients with chronic AR, preserved LVEF and non-dilated LVs, global longitudinal strain values worse than −19% were associated with increased 5-year all-cause mortality. [21] Global longitudinal strain also provides prognostic value in patients with AR who undergo surgery. For example, within a cohort of patients with severe chronic AR who underwent surgical aortic valve replacement (AVR) or repair, global longitudinal strain values worse than −19% were again associated with increased 5-year mortality. [22] Importantly, patients in this cohort who had persistently low global longitudinal strain values post-surgery had the highest mortality rates. [22] Therefore, the addition of global longitudinal strain to a 2D TTE may certainly provide important diagnostic and prognostic information in all patients with AR.

Cardiac MRI

Through analysis of LV volume, LV function, and flow dynamics across the AV, cardiac magnetic resonance (CMR) is an effective and comprehensive method of evaluating AR. Due to the direct aortic measurements obtained during phase contrast imaging, CMR quantifies regurgitant volume in patients with AR by determining antegrade and retrograde flow at the sinotubular junction. [23–25] Through these measurements, the AV regurgitant volume and regurgitant fraction may be calculated with high degrees of sensitivity and with greater accuracy than that achieved by echocardiography. [23]

In addition to assessing the AV directly, CMR also measures flow reversal in the descending aorta to provide a comprehensive analysis of AR severity in affected individuals. [23] Detection of descending aortic flow reversal can be further enhanced by 4-dimensional flow MRI. [26]

CMR is uniquely well suited to evaluate AR-HF due to enhanced identification of abnormal LV structure and function. Through superior delineation between blood and myocardium, CMR allows for reproducible measurements of LV volume, mass, and ejection fraction. [24] Indeed, prior work has demonstrated that CMR provides more reproducible data on LV volume and LVEF than TTE. [27] Furthermore, CMR detects myocardial fibrosis, which is inherent to the pathogenesis of LV dysfunction in severe AR, and is strongly associated with incident HF syndromes. [28,29]

As a result of the 3D measurements obtained, improved interrater reliability, and accurate quantification of LV volumes, CMR provides a more precise estimation of LVEF, LV end-diastolic and end-systolic volumes, and regurgitant volume, than TTE. [24,30] Furthermore, CMR does not rely on patients having adequate sonographic windows to obtain images. Particularly in patients who have undergone prior valve replacement, or have oblique regurgitant jets, CMR may provide incremental benefit over TTE for evaluation of AR. [24] Accordingly, both the American College of Cardiology (ACC)/American Heart Association (AHA) and European Society of Cardiology (ESC) guidelines recommend the use of CMR to assess AR when TTE views are inadequate. [3,31] Additionally, CMR carries a Class I recommendation for assessment of LV volume, function, and AR severity once AR has been diagnosed. [3,31]

Another advantage of CMR is the detailed interrogation of the ascending aorta. A significant percentage of patients with AR, particularly those with bicuspid aortic valves, have concomitant aortopathy, and CMR is uniquely well suited to simultaneously evaluate AR and the ascending aorta in affected individuals. [32] Accordingly, CMR is a guideline-recommended imaging modality in patients with AR who have bicuspid AV disease or have known aortic dilation with diameters >4 cm. [3]

In addition to characterizing AR, CMR may provide significant prognostic data in patients with AR. [23,33] For example, within a cohort of 232 patients, CMR-derived holosystolic retrograde flow in patients with AR was associated with subsequent progression to clinical HF, cardiovascular death, and hospitalization. [23] Furthermore, in a separate cohort of 178 patients with moderate or severe AR without clinical HF, CMR derived LV end-systolic volume index LVESVi greater than 45 mL/m^2 and aortic regurgitant fraction greater than 31% were both associated with the development of incident HF. [33] Indeed, additional small studies demonstrate that CMR is superior to TTE in predicting which patients with AR ultimately progress to clinical HF and AV surgery. [34]

Limitations of cardiac magnetic resonance

Although CMR provides more reproducible data on AV parameters than TTE, quantification of AR by CMR relies on the assumption that the imaging plane is perpendicular to the regurgitant flow, which may be difficult when highly eccentric jets are present. Accordingly, altering the slice of measurement may result in significant changes to calculated forward and regurgitant stroke volumes, and subsequently alter AR classification. [35] In addition, CMR reliability is limited in patients with arrhythmia, due to the need for regular R-R intervals to accurately calculate valve parameters. [24] Compared to TTE, CMR is associated with higher costs and reduced availability. Finally, patients with claustrophobia may not tolerate the prolonged scan time needed for CMR. [24]

Transesophageal Echocardiography

Transesophageal echocardiography (TEE) is an additional imaging modality that provides valuable information for the characterization of AR. TEE may be particularly useful when TTE is limited by suboptimal windows, or when descending aortic pathology needs to be evaluated. Compared to TTE, TEE increases diagnostic accuracy in determining the etiology and severity of AR, particularly when there are highly eccentric regurgitant jets.[36–38] As a result of this increased ability to determine the etiology of AR, intraoperative TEE may provide valuable information regarding the ability for an AV to be repaired, rather than replaced, at the time of surgery. [38]

Unlike TTE and CMR, TEE does not provide detail on LV myocardial function. Accordingly, TEE is limited in its assessment of impaired LV function and HF associated with AR, compared to alternate imaging modalities. In addition, TEE is an invasive procedure, and therefore, may not be suitable for all AR patients.

Cardiac Catheterization

Cardiac catheterization provides semi-quantitative assessment of AR severity by assessing the degree of LV opacification after contrast injection into the proximal aorta. Furthermore, LV cineangiography allows for the measurement of LV volumes and LVEF with high degrees of correlation to TTE.[6,39,40] Therefore, cardiac catheterization provides both functional information about the degree of AR and downstream consequences on LVEF.

Cardiac catheterization may be beneficial in circumstances in which noninvasive tests produce discrepant results and 3D imaging is not available or prohibitive due to comorbidities. However, due to the increasing availability and tolerance of advanced noninvasive imaging techniques, cardiac catheterization is rarely used for the contemporary assessment of AR.[6]

Laboratory Assessment

B-type natriuretic peptide (BNP) is released by cardiac myocytes in response to increased mechanical stretch. Numerous studies have assessed associations between BNP and AR clinical outcomes with conflicting results.[41,42] Although certain studies have not established a correlation between BNP and the degree of LV dysfunction among patients with AR, others have suggested that among a subgroup of patients with severe AR and normal LV systolic function, BNP greater than 130 pg/mL is associated with eventual progression to reduced LVEF and HF symptoms.[41,42] Accordingly, BNP may be used as a component of a comprehensive AR evaluation, but should not be used in isolation to predict AR-HF outcomes.

MANAGEMENT

In this section, we will review management strategies for those with, or at risk for, AR-HF. There is no convincing evidence that medical therapy has value in asymptomatic patients in preventing progression to LV dysfunction and/or symptoms.[3] The only effective treatment of patients with symptomatic AR, or those with severe LV dilation or reduced LVEF at risk for AR-HF, is operative management. Symptomatic patients considered to have a prohibitive risk for surgical AVR due to age or comorbidities are candidates for guideline-directed medical therapy for HF for symptomatic improvement. As will be detailed, some patients who are not candidates for surgical AVR may benefit from off-label transcatheter-based therapies, based on recent advances in the literature.

Medical Management

Among patients with severe AR who have not yet progressed to HF, long-term afterload-reducing therapies have not been shown to decrease the regurgitant volume and slow the progression of LV dilation and systolic dysfunction. However, guidelines do recommend treating hypertension (SBP>140 mm Hg) in patients with AR, as with other patients with hypertension.[3] It should be recognized that elevation of systolic blood pressure is common in patients with severe AR due to the elevated forward stroke volume, and it is often difficult to normalize blood pressure even with multiple anti-hypertensive medications that may only result in drug side effects.

Surgical Aortic Valve Replacement

Surgical AVR has been the mainstay of management for severe AR to reduce the rates of AR-HF and LV dysfunction in appropriate patients.[43] A significant percentage of AR patients ultimately meet indications for AVR.[44] Within cohorts of asymptomatic patients with severe AR and preserved LVEF, 2% to 6% progress to impaired LVEF or clinical HF necessitating surgery per year.[45–48] However, the frequency of progression to symptomatic HF is related to the degree of existing LV dilation and/or dysfunction. In fact, among patients with LV end-systolic diameter of greater than 50 mm by 2D TTE, ~20% may progress to symptomatic HF and LV dysfunction per year.[5] Additional risk factors for progression to AR-HF include LV end-systolic dimension index (LVESDi) > 25 mm/m^2 and LVESVi greater than 45 mL/m.[2,11,25,33,49]

Among patients with AR and impaired LVEF, the duration of time of LV dysfunction is inversely related to the probability of LVEF recovery following AVR,[50] and impaired systolic function is a risk factor for poor outcomes after AVR.[3,51,52] These findings are likely due to the interstitial fibrosis and cellular remodeling associated with LV dysfunction and support indications for operative intervention before onset of myocardial dysfunction and clinical HF.[3,6] Indeed, current guidelines combine AR characteristics, symptoms, and LV structure/function to make recommendations on appropriateness and timing for AVR (**Fig. 2**).[3]

Patients with symptomatic severe AR should undergo AVR. Additionally, to prevent the development of AR-HF, contemporary guidelines recommend that asymptomatic patients with severe AR and impaired LV systolic function (LVEF $\leq$55% or LVESD >50 mm [or LVESDi >25 mm/m^2] by 2D TTE) should undergo AVR.[3] Conversely, those with severe asymptomatic AR, and preserved LVEF and LV dimensions, can be monitored closely for disease progression.[3,46] It should be noted that the current recommended threshold of LVESDi of 25 mm/m^2 for AVR in asymptomatic patients may be set too high, as recent studies report the risk of adverse

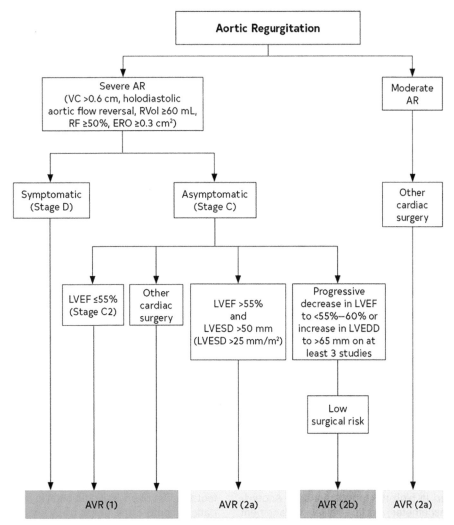

Fig. 2. Guideline-directed management of AR. Guideline recommended treatment thresholds for surgical AVR in patients with aortic regurgitation. AR, aortic regurgitation; AVR, aortic valve replacement; LVEDD, left ventricular end-diastolic diameter; LVEF, left ventricular ejection fraction; LVESD, left ventricular end-systolic diameter. (Otto C, Nishimura R, et al. 2020 ACC/AHA Guideline for the Management of Patients With Valvular Heart Disease. J Am Coll Cardiol. 2021 Feb, 77 (4) e25–e197. https://doi.org/10.1016/j.jacc.2020.11.018.)

outcomes, including death and AR-HF, at levels of LVESDi as low as 20 to 22 mm/m^2, suggesting earlier intervention may improve outcomes.[53–55] Indeed, recent volumetric data from TTE and CMR indicate adverse event rates in asymptomatic patients with LVESVi greater than 45 mL/m.[2,11,25,33,56] Furthermore, cohort studies have reported that regurgitant fraction thresholds for severe AR may be different by CMR than by TTE, with the CMR threshold lower than what is reported in current guidelines.[57]

The decision for AVR using a mechanical prosthesis versus a bioprosthesis is a complex decision between clinician and patient regarding the tradeoffs of lifelong anticoagulation versus prosthesis durability. The variable durability of surgically implanted bioprosthetic valves may necessitate repeated procedures across the lifespan.[58] This is particularly relevant for patients undergoing surgery for bicuspid AV, who tend to be young. In these cases, AVR with a mechanical valve may be preferable. However, AV repair may be an appealing option when AV anatomy permits, with increased longevity compared to AVR in appropriately selected populations referred to centers that are experts in repair.[59–61] In addition, the Ross procedure, in which the AV is replaced by a pulmonary valve autograft, and the pulmonary valve replaced by a homograft or xenograft, has shown a recent resurgence in the surgical management of AR.[61] Due to the potential for long-term autograft dilation, modifications to the Ross procedure, which provide additional support to the ascending aorta, have been proposed.[62] Indeed, the Ross procedure, with or without modifications, may be a particularly attractive option in young patients, who seek to avoid prolonged exposure to anticoagulation or repeat sternotomies, and in expert centers has excellent long-term durability.[63–65]

TRANSCATHETER AORTIC VALVE REPLACEMENT

Despite meeting guideline indications for surgery, an analysis of the Euro Heart Survey recently disclosed that only ~20% of patients with severe AR and LVEF 30% to 50% were referred for surgery, and ~3% of patients with severe AR and LVEF less than 30% proceeded to AVR.[66] This is likely due to the morbidity associated with surgery, which is magnified in high-risk populations.[66] Accordingly, transcatheter aortic valve replacement (TAVR) has been investigated as an alternative to surgical AVR in high-risk patients with severe AR.

Before recent advancements, AR has proven to be a difficult physiology for TAVR. Unlike patients with severe aortic stenosis, many patients with severe AR do not have annular calcification to anchor the TAVR valve. In addition, patients with AR often have annular dilation that necessitates implantation of a large or oversized valve.[67]

Recently, TAVR has emerged as an off-label alternative to surgical AVR for select patients with AR who meet indications for surgery. As TAVR technology has progressed to encompass valves that can be repositioned and have superior fixation methods, implantation of TAVR in a non-calcified and dilated aortic annulus has become technically possible.[67,68] Indeed, newer generation valves have demonstrated superiority to earlier designs with respect to endpoints including successful deployment and residual AR.[69] Strategies employed to increase rates of successful deployment include valve oversizing, utilization of a valve that incorporates anchors superior or inferior to the annulus, or a clip fixation system.[69] Although not currently guideline recommended or approved by the United States Food and Drug Administration, select centers have shown feasibility of TAVR in non-calcified severe AR-HF.[69,70]

Results following TAVR for severe AR are variable. In a large single study of 134 patients who underwent TAVR for AR, average LVEF increased significantly from 52.1% to 57.1% and pulmonary arterial pressures decreased to the normal range by 30 days post-procedure. However, within this cohort, 3.7% required conversion to an open procedure, and 30-day mortality was 3%.[70] A systematic review of 10 studies investigating TAVR for AR revealed successful valve deployment in 70% to 100% of patients, coupled with 9% all-cause mortality by 30-days post-procedure.[69] Due to the need for valve oversizing, conduction abnormalities are a theoretic risk following TAVR for AR that should be investigated further. Currently, the JenaValve ALIGN-AR Pivotal Trial (NCT04415047) is ongoing to systematically assess the safety and efficacy of a novel TAVR valve in patients with severe, symptomatic AR.

SUMMARY

In this review, we discussed the evaluation and management of AR-HF. Although the review is focused on AR-HF, HF exists on the spectrum of AR severity. Accordingly, the diagnostic methods discussed should be used to detect AR and its effects on LV volumes and function in asymptomatic patients before the onset of LV dysfunction and clinical HF.

Recently, advances in imaging modalities via speckle tracking echocardiography, 3D echocardiography, and CMR have enhanced the ability to detect early signs of HF in patients with AR.

Although many of these imaging modalities are not yet incorporated into guidelines, specific cohorts of patients may benefit from early detection of AR to potentially prevent incident HF. Further studies validating the prognostic value of these advanced imaging techniques, and thresholds for intervention, are needed.

Furthermore, whereas surgical AVR has remained the only guideline-recommended option for intervention for severe AR, many patients with severe AR or AR-HF are not candidates for surgery due to age and comorbidities. Forthcoming trial data on utility of TAVR in severe symptomatic AR may expand treatment options for such patients in the future. If shown to be effective, further efforts are required to identify patients who would benefit most from transcatheter-based therapies for AR.

CLINICS CARE POINTS

- Assessing for subclinical signs of HF may impact treatment decisions in patients with AR.

- 2D transthoracic echocardiography is the mainstay of evaluation for patients with AR, however, additional imaging techniques including speckle tracking echocardiography, 3D echocardiography, and cardiac MRI can provide important diagnostic and prognostic information.

- The only effective treatment of patients with symptomatic AR, or those with AR and left ventricular dilation or reduced LVEF, is operative management.

- Surgical AVR is the primary operative procedure for AR, however, when evaluating patients with AR, it is important to consider AV repair or the Ross procedure in appropriate clinical settings.

- Data are forthcoming on the safety and efficacy of TAVR in patients with AR who meet indications for AVR, but are not operative candidates.

DISCLOSURE

The authors have nothing to disclose. This research did not receive any specific grant from funding agencies in the public, commercial, or not-for-profit sectors.

ACKNOWLEDGMENT

The Central Illustration was created on biorender. com

REFERENCES

1. Singh JP, Evans JC, Levy D, et al. Prevalence and clinical determinants of mitral, tricuspid, and aortic regurgitation (the Framingham Heart Study). Am J Cardiol 1999;83(6):897–902.
2. Maurer G. Aortic regurgitation. Heart 2006;92(7): 994–1000.
3. Otto CM, Nishimura RA, Bonow RO, et al. 2020 ACC/ AHA Guideline for the Management of Patients With Valvular Heart Disease: A Report of the American College of Cardiology/American Heart Association Joint Committee on Clinical Practice Guidelines. Circulation 2021;143(5):e72–227.
4. Peter CA, Jones RH. Cardiac response to exercise in patients with chronic aortic regurgitation. Am Heart J 1982;104(1):85–91.
5. Bonow RONR. Aortic regurgitation. In: Libby PBR, Mann DL, Tommaselli GF, et al, editors. Braunwald's heart disease. A Textbook of cardiovascular medicine. 12 edition. Philadelphia, PA: Elsevier; 2020. p. 1419–29.
6. Akinseye OA, Pathak A, Ibebuogu UN. Aortic Valve Regurgitation: A Comprehensive Review. Curr Probl Cardiol 2018;43(8):315–34.
7. Chambers J. Aortic Regurgitation: The Value of Clinical Signs. J Am Coll Cardiol 2020;75(1):40–1.
8. Mehta M, Jacobson T, Peters D, et al. Handheld ultrasound versus physical examination in patients referred for transthoracic echocardiography for a suspected cardiac condition. JACC Cardiovasc Imaging 2014;7(10):983–90.
9. Lancellotti P, Tribouilloy C, Hagendorff A, et al. Recommendations for the echocardiographic assessment of native valvular regurgitation: an executive summary from the European Association of Cardiovascular Imaging. Eur Heart J Cardiovasc Imaging 2013;14(7):611–44.
10. Zoghbi WA, Adams D, Bonow RO, et al. Recommendations for Noninvasive Evaluation of Native Valvular Regurgitation: A Report from the American Society of Echocardiography Developed in Collaboration with the Society for Cardiovascular Magnetic Resonance. J Am Soc Echocardiogr 2017;30(4):303–71.
11. Yang LT, Anand V, Zambito EI, et al. Association of Echocardiographic Left Ventricular End-Systolic Volume and Volume-Derived Ejection Fraction With Outcome in Asymptomatic Chronic Aortic Regurgitation. JAMA Cardiol 2021;6(2):189–98.
12. Hagendorff A, Evangelista A, Fehske W, et al. Improvement in the Assessment of Aortic Valve and Aortic Aneurysm Repair by 3-Dimensional Echocardiography. JACC Cardiovasc Imaging 2019;12(11 Pt 1):2225–44.
13. Ewe SH, Delgado V, van der Geest R, et al. Accuracy of three-dimensional versus two-dimensional echocardiography for quantification of aortic regurgitation and validation by three-dimensional three-

directional velocity-encoded magnetic resonance imaging. Am J Cardiol 2013;112(4):560–6.

14. Vaidya GN, Salgado BC, Badar F, et al. Two-dimensional strain echocardiography-derived left ventricular ejection fraction, volumes, and global systolic dyssynchrony index: Comparison with three-dimensional echocardiography. Echocardiography 2019;36(6):1054–65.

15. Peigh G, Shah SJ, Patel RB. Left Atrial Myopathy in Atrial Fibrillation and Heart Failure: Clinical Implications, Mechanisms, and Therapeutic Targets. Curr Heart Fail Rep 2021;18(3):85–98.

16. Cavalcante JL. Global Longitudinal Strain in Asymptomatic Chronic Aortic Regurgitation: The Missing Piece for the Watchful Waiting Puzzle? JACC Cardiovasc Imaging 2018;11(5):683–5.

17. Mizariene V, Bucyte S, Zaliaduonyte-Peksiene D, et al. Left ventricular mechanics in asymptomatic normotensive and hypertensive patients with aortic regurgitation. J Am Soc Echocardiogr 2011;24(4): 385–91.

18. Kaneko A, Tanaka H, Onishi T, et al. Subendocardial dysfunction in patients with chronic severe aortic regurgitation and preserved ejection fraction detected with speckle-tracking strain imaging and transmural myocardial strain profile. Eur Heart J Cardiovasc Imaging 2013;14(4):339–46.

19. Smedsrud MK, Pettersen E, Gjesdal O, et al. Detection of left ventricular dysfunction by global longitudinal systolic strain in patients with chronic aortic regurgitation. J Am Soc Echocardiogr 2011;24(11): 1253–9.

20. Di Salvo G, Pacileo G, Verrengia M, et al. Early myocardial abnormalities in asymptomatic patients with severe isolated congenital aortic regurgitation: an ultrasound tissue characterization and strain rate study. J Am Soc Echocardiogr 2005;18(2):122–7.

21. Alashi A, Mentias A, Abdallah A, et al. Incremental Prognostic Utility of Left Ventricular Global Longitudinal Strain in Asymptomatic Patients With Significant Chronic Aortic Regurgitation and Preserved Left Ventricular Ejection Fraction. JACC Cardiovasc Imaging 2018;11(5):673–82.

22. Alashi A, Khullar T, Mentias A, et al. Long-Term Outcomes After Aortic Valve Surgery in Patients With Asymptomatic Chronic Aortic Regurgitation and Preserved LVEF: Impact of Baseline and Follow-Up Global Longitudinal Strain. JACC Cardiovasc Imaging 2020;13(1 Pt 1):12–21.

23. Kammerlander AA, Wiesinger M, Duca F, et al. Diagnostic and Prognostic Utility of Cardiac Magnetic Resonance Imaging in Aortic Regurgitation. JACC Cardiovasc Imaging 2019;12(8 Pt 1):1474–83.

24. Lee JC, Branch KR, Hamilton-Craig C, et al. Evaluation of aortic regurgitation with cardiac magnetic resonance imaging: a systematic review. Heart 2018;104(2):103–10.

25. Myerson SG, d'Arcy J, Mohiaddin R, et al. Aortic regurgitation quantification using cardiovascular magnetic resonance: association with clinical outcome. Circulation 2012;126(12):1452–60.

26. Mor-Avi V, Jenkins C, Kuhl HP, et al. Real-time 3-dimensional echocardiographic quantification of left ventricular volumes: multicenter study for validation with magnetic resonance imaging and investigation of sources of error. JACC Cardiovasc Imaging 2008;1(4):413–23.

27. Grothues F, Smith GC, Moon JC, et al. Comparison of interstudy reproducibility of cardiovascular magnetic resonance with two-dimensional echocardiography in normal subjects and in patients with heart failure or left ventricular hypertrophy. Am J Cardiol 2002;90(1):29–34.

28. Sparrow P, Messroghli DR, Reid S, et al. Myocardial T1 mapping for detection of left ventricular myocardial fibrosis in chronic aortic regurgitation: pilot study. AJR Am J Roentgenol 2006;187(6):W630–5.

29. Senapati A, Malahfji M, Debs D, et al. Regional Replacement and Diffuse Interstitial Fibrosis in Aortic Regurgitation: Prognostic Implications From Cardiac Magnetic Resonance. JACC Cardiovasc Imaging 2021;14(11):2170–82.

30. Cawley PJ, Hamilton-Craig C, Owens DS, et al. Prospective comparison of valve regurgitation quantitation by cardiac magnetic resonance imaging and transthoracic echocardiography. Circ Cardiovasc Imaging 2013;6(1):48–57.

31. Baumgartner H, Falk V, Bax JJ, et al. 2017 ESC/EACTS Guidelines for the management of valvular heart disease. Eur Heart J 2017;38(36):2739–91.

32. Popovic ZB, Desai MY, Griffin BP. Decision Making With Imaging in Asymptomatic Aortic Regurgitation. JACC Cardiovasc Imaging 2018;11(10):1499–513.

33. Hashimoto G, Enriquez-Sarano M, Stanberry LI, et al. Association of Left Ventricular Remodeling Assessment by Cardiac Magnetic Resonance With Outcomes in Patients With Chronic Aortic Regurgitation. JAMA Cardiol 2022;7(9):924–33.

34. Harris AW, Krieger EV, Kim M, et al. Cardiac Magnetic Resonance Imaging Versus Transthoracic Echocardiography for Prediction of Outcomes in Chronic Aortic or Mitral Regurgitation. Am J Cardiol 2017;119(7):1074–81.

35. Chaturvedi A, Hamilton-Craig C, Cawley PJ, et al. Quantitating aortic regurgitation by cardiovascular magnetic resonance: significant variations due to slice location and breath holding. Eur Radiol 2016; 26(9):3180–9.

36. La Canna G, Maisano F, De Michele L, et al. Determinants of the degree of functional aortic regurgitation in patients with anatomically normal aortic valve and ascending thoracic aorta aneurysm. Transoesophageal Doppler echocardiography study. Heart 2009;95(2):130–6.

37. American College of Cardiology Foundation Appropriate Use Criteria Task F, American Society of E, American Heart A, et al. ACCF/ASE/AHA/ASNC/HFSA/HRS/SCAI/SCCM/SCCT/SCMR 2011 Appropriate Use Criteria for Echocardiography. A Report of the American College of Cardiology Foundation Appropriate Use Criteria Task Force, American Society of Echocardiography, American Heart Association, American Society of Nuclear Cardiology, Heart Failure Society of America, Heart Rhythm Society, Society for Cardiovascular Angiography and Interventions, Society of Critical Care Medicine, Society of Cardiovascular Computed Tomography, Society for Cardiovascular Magnetic Resonance American College of Chest Physicians. J Am Soc Echocardiogr 2011;24(3):229–67.

38. le Polain de Waroux JB, Pouleur AC, Goffinet C, et al. Functional anatomy of aortic regurgitation: accuracy, prediction of surgical repairability, and outcome implications of transesophageal echocardiography. Circulation 2007;116(11 Suppl):I264–9.

39. Griffin B, Callahan TD, Menon V, et al. Valvular Heart Disease. In: Manual of cardiovascular medicine, vol 1, 4 edition. Philadelphia PA: Lippincott Williams & Wilkins; 2013. p. 238–355.

40. Bonow RO, Borer JS, Rosing DR, et al. Preoperative exercise capacity in symptomatic patients with aortic regurgitation as a predictor of postoperative left ventricular function and long-term prognosis. Circulation 1980;62(6):1280–90.

41. Pizarro R, Bazzino OO, Oberti PF, et al. Prospective validation of the prognostic usefulness of B-type natriuretic peptide in asymptomatic patients with chronic severe aortic regurgitation. J Am Coll Cardiol 2011;58(16):1705–14.

42. Eimer MJ, Ekery DL, Rigolin VH, et al. Elevated B-type natriuretic peptide in asymptomatic men with chronic aortic regurgitation and preserved left ventricular systolic function. Am J Cardiol 2004; 94(5):676–8.

43. Detaint D, Maalouf J, Tribouilloy C, et al. Congestive heart failure complicating aortic regurgitation with medical and surgical management: a prospective study of traditional and quantitative echocardiographic markers. J Thorac Cardiovasc Surg 2008; 136(6):1549–57.

44. Yang LT, Lo HY, Lee CC, et al. Comparison Between Bicuspid and Tricuspid Aortic Regurgitation: Presentation, Survival, and Aorta Complications. JACC Asia 2022;2(4):476–86.

45. Tornos MP, Olona M, Permanyer-Miralda G, et al. Clinical outcome of severe asymptomatic chronic aortic regurgitation: a long-term prospective follow-up study. Am Heart J 1995;130(2):333–9.

46. Bonow RO, Lakatos E, Maron BJ, et al. Serial long-term assessment of the natural history of asymptomatic patients with chronic aortic regurgitation and

47. Siemienczuk D, Greenberg B, Morris C, et al. Chronic aortic insufficiency: factors associated with progression to aortic valve replacement. Ann Intern Med 1989;110(8):587–92.

48. Bonow RO, Rosing DR, McIntosh CL, et al. The natural history of asymptomatic patients with aortic regurgitation and normal left ventricular function. Circulation 1983;68(3).

49. Dujardin KS, Enriquez-Sarano M, Schaff HV, et al. Mortality and morbidity of aortic regurgitation in clinical practice. A long-term follow-up study. Circulation 1999;99(14):1851–7.

50. Bonow RO, Picone AL, McIntosh CL, et al. Survival and functional results after valve replacement for aortic regurgitation from 1976 to 1983: impact of preoperative left ventricular function. Circulation 1985;72(6):1244–56.

51. Murashita T, Schaff HV, Suri RM, et al. Impact of Left Ventricular Systolic Function on Outcome of Correction of Chronic Severe Aortic Valve Regurgitation: Implications for Timing of Surgical Intervention. Ann Thorac Surg 2017;103(4):1222–8.

52. Anand V, Nishimura RA, Rigolin VH. Earlier Intervention in Asymptomatic Chronic Aortic Regurgitation-Novel Indicators of Myocardial Overload. JAMA Cardiol 2022;7(9):883–4.

53. de Meester C, Gerber BL, Vancraeynest D, et al. Do Guideline-Based Indications Result in an Outcome Penalty for Patients With Severe Aortic Regurgitation? JACC Cardiovasc Imaging 2019;12(11 Pt 1): 2126–38.

54. Mentias A, Feng K, Alashi A, et al. Long-Term Outcomes in Patients With Aortic Regurgitation and Preserved Left Ventricular Ejection Fraction. J Am Coll Cardiol 2016;68(20):2144–53.

55. Yang LT, Michelena HI, Scott CG, et al. Outcomes in Chronic Hemodynamically Significant Aortic Regurgitation and Limitations of Current Guidelines. J Am Coll Cardiol 2019;73(14):1741–52.

56. Bonow RO, O'Gara PT. Left Ventricular Volume and Outcomes in Patients With Chronic Aortic Regurgitation. JAMA Cardiol 2022;7(9):885–6.

57. Vejpongsa P, Xu J, Quinones MA, et al. Differences in Cardiac Remodeling in Left-Sided Valvular Regurgitation: Implications for Optimal Definition of Significant Aortic Regurgitation. JACC Cardiovasc Imaging 2022;15(10):1730–41.

58. Flint N, Wunderlich NC, Shmueli H, et al. Aortic Regurgitation. Curr Cardiol Rep 2019;21(7):65.

59. Kari FA, Siepe M, Sievers HH, et al. Repair of the regurgitant bicuspid or tricuspid aortic valve: background, principles, and outcomes. Circulation 2013;128(8):854–63.

60. Schneider U, Hofmann C, Schope J, et al. Long-term Results of Differentiated Anatomic Reconstruction of

normal left ventricular systolic function. Circulation 1991;84(4):1625–35.

Bicuspid Aortic Valves. JAMA Cardiol 2020;5(12): 1366–73.

61. Baman JR, Medhekar AN, Malaisrie SC, et al. Management Challenges in Patients Younger Than 65 Years With Severe Aortic Valve Disease: A Review. JAMA Cardiol 2022. https://doi.org/10.1001/jamacardio.2022.4770.

62. Abeln KB, Schafers S, Ehrlich T, et al. Ross Operation With Autologous External Autograft Stabilization-Long-term Results. Ann Thorac Surg 2022;114(2): 502–9.

63. El-Hamamsy I, Warnes CA, Nishimura RA. The Ross Procedure in Adults: The Ideal Aortic Valve Substitute? J Am Coll Cardiol 2021;77(11):1423–5.

64. Mazine A, El-Hamamsy I. The Ross procedure is an excellent operation in non-repairable aortic regurgitation: insights and techniques. Ann Cardiothorac Surg 2021;10(4):463–75.

65. Mazine A, El-Hamamsy I, Verma S, et al. Ross Procedure in Adults for Cardiologists and Cardiac Surgeons: JACC State-of-the-Art Review. J Am Coll Cardiol 2018;72(22):2761–77.

66. Iung B, Baron G, Butchart EG, et al. A prospective survey of patients with valvular heart disease in Europe: The Euro Heart Survey on Valvular Heart Disease. Eur Heart J 2003;24(13):1231–43.

67. Franzone A, Piccolo R, Siontis GCM, et al. Transcatheter Aortic Valve Replacement for the Treatment of Pure Native Aortic Valve Regurgitation: A Systematic Review. JACC Cardiovasc Interv 2016;9(22): 2308–17.

68. Pesarini G, Lunardi M, Piccoli A, et al. Effectiveness and Safety of Transcatheter Aortic Valve Implantation in Patients With Pure Aortic Regurgitation and Advanced Heart Failure. Am J Cardiol 2018;121(5): 642–8.

69. Jiang J, Liu X, He Y, et al. Transcatheter Aortic Valve Replacement for Pure Native Aortic Valve Regurgitation: A Systematic Review. Cardiology 2018;141(3): 132–40.

70. Liu L, Chen S, Shi J, et al. Transcatheter Aortic Valve Replacement in Aortic Regurgitation. Ann Thorac Surg 2020;110(6):1959–65.

Primary Mitral Regurgitation and Heart Failure
Current Advances in Diagnosis and Management

Brody Slostad, MD, Gloria Ayuba, DO, Jyothy J. Puthumana, MD*

KEYWORDS

- Primary mitral regurgitation • Myxomatous mitral valve • Heart failure • Outcomes
- Transcatheter edge-to-edge repair

KEY POINTS

- Severe primary mitral regurgitation is associated with excess mortality and heart failure morbidity when left untreated.
- Patients with severe primary mitral regurgitation with no symptoms and normal left ventricular parameters exhibit an increase in adverse outcomes.
- Early surgical or transcatheter mitral valve intervention can improve outcomes substantially.
- Despite improvement in outcomes with mitral valve intervention, only a small proportion of patients ultimately receive this therapy.
- There are increasing options for transcatheter therapy with ongoing studies to apply these less invasive therapies to moderate and low surgical risk patients. This ideally will improve the undertreatment of primary mitral regurgitation.

INTRODUCTION

Congestive heart failure is often accompanied by mitral valve disease, in particular, mitral regurgitation. Mitral regurgitation is the most frequently diagnosed moderate or severe valvular heart disease with an estimated prevalence of 9% in individuals aged 75 years and older and a total prevalence of 13% in the general population.[1] The mitral valve apparatus is complex and includes the leaflets, papillary muscles, and chordae. Problems with any subcomponent of the apparatus may result in mitral regurgitation.[2] Primary mitral regurgitation is caused by a fundamental abnormality of the mitral valve apparatus leading to mitral regurgitation and is the focus of this review. The natural history of severe mitral regurgitation leads to poor cardiovascular outcomes including heart failure symptoms, hospitalizations, and mortality. However, early intervention with surgical or transcatheter techniques can improve outcomes substantially.[3–6] Accordingly, over 30,000 mitral valve surgeries are performed each year, with most of these surgeries being performed for the indication of mitral regurgitation.[7] Given the importance of early detection, the purpose of this review is to highlight current advances in diagnosis and treatment of primary mitral regurgitation.

PRIMARY MITRAL REGURGITATION

Primary mitral regurgitation is defined as a fundamental abnormality of the mitral valve apparatus. The most frequent source of primary mitral

Bluhm Cardiovascular Institute, Northwestern University, 675 North St Clair Street Ste 19-100, Galter Pavilion, Chicago, IL 60611, USA
* Corresponding author.
E-mail address: jyothy.puthumana@nm.org

Heart Failure Clin 19 (2023) 297–305
https://doi.org/10.1016/j.hfc.2023.02.006
1551-7136/23/© 2023 Elsevier Inc. All rights reserved.

heartfailure.theclinics.com

regurgitation is mitral valve prolapse as a result of myxomatous degeneration or fibroelastic deficiency.[8] Fibroelastic deficiency typically presents with fine leaflets and associated focal prolapse, chordal rupture, or flail. Whereas, myxomatous degeneration such as with Barlow's disease typically presents with redundant leaflet tissue that becomes stretched or torn leading to prolapse or flail (**Fig. 1**).[8,9] Less frequent causes of primary mitral regurgitation include endocarditis, prior radiation exposure, congenital heart disease, and mitral annular calcification.[10]

NATURAL HISTORY

Primary mitral regurgitation natural history studies have focused on those patients with mitral valve prolapse or flail mitral leaflet. Early studies of mitral valve prolapse showed an overall and cardiovascular mortality at 5 years from initial diagnosis at 19% and 9%, respectively.[11] Mitral valve prolapse-related cardiovascular events (including death or heart failure) occurred in 20% of these patients, with 8% of patients ultimately requiring mitral valve surgery.[11] In this early study, risk factors for cardiovascular mortality in patients diagnosed with mitral valve prolapse were also investigated. This revealed that the key risk factor for worse outcomes was moderate to severe mitral regurgitation.

Other early studies have similarly shown that the severity of mitral regurgitation predicts mitral valve prolapse-associated morbidity and mortality.[12] Further identified independent risk factors for morbidity and mortality were left ventricular ejection fraction (LVEF) less than 50%, left atrial enlargement, atrial fibrillation, age $\geq$ 50 years,

and presence of flail leaflet.[12] Later studies specifically looking at more precise quantification of mitral regurgitation revealed that an effective regurgitant orifice area (EROA) $\geq$ 40 mm^2 predicts worse outcomes.[3] The duration of mitral regurgitation with respect to the cardiac cycle is also important for predicting outcomes, especially in cases of mitral valve prolapse where the mitral regurgitation may be holosystolic or mid to late systolic with considerable variations in resultant regurgitant volumes.[13]

A subset of patients with primary mitral regurgitation caused by mitral valve prolapse may also present with mitral annular disjunction. Mitral annular disjunction is a malformation of the mitral annulus fibrosus which produces a systolic aperture at the basal inferolateral myocardium at the site of the posterior mitral valve leaflet insertion.[14] This subset of patients is at risk of developing progressive left ventricular dilatation and ventricular arrhythmias.[14]

Primary mitral regurgitation natural history studies have also focused on those patients with flail leaflet specifically. Mitral regurgitation tends to advance more precipitously in the presence of flail mitral leaflet. This has been shown in multiple studies of mitral valve prolapse in which patients also diagnosed with flail leaflet had more rapid evolution of worsening mitral regurgitation severity compared to those without flail.[15,16] Long-term outcomes of patients with flail mitral leaflet showed that at 10 years, 90% of patients had undergone mitral valve surgery or were deceased with risk factors for decreased survival and worsening mitral regurgitation in this cohort including New York Heart Association (NYHA) class III or

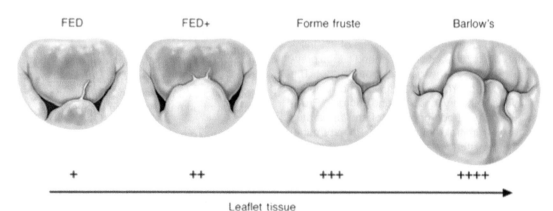

Fig. 1. Primary mitral regurgitation most commonly results from fibroelastic deficiency or myxomatous degeneration. Fibroelastic deficiency results from a paucity of collagen most often leading to ruptured chordae. Whereas, myxomatous degeneration results from redundant leaflets leading to stretching and rupture or one or multiple chordae and ultimately mitral valve prolapse or flail. Excessively redundant tissue resulting in myxomatous disease is termed Barlow's disease. (*From* Adams DH, Rosenhek R, Falk V. Degenerative mitral valve regurgitation: best practice revolution. *Eur Heart J.* 2010;31(16):1958 to 1966.)

IV symptoms and LVEF less than 60%. Subsequent studies have demonstrated survival benefit in those receiving mitral valve surgery which highlights the importance of early diagnosis to allow for improved outcomes.[16–18]

CLINICAL PRESENTATION AND DIAGNOSIS

Patients with chronic primary mitral regurgitation may not develop symptoms for several years due to gradual remodeling and offsetting left ventricular dilatation.[19] Once these compensatory mechanisms are overcome from worsening volume overload from mitral regurgitation, symptoms such as dyspnea on exertion, orthopnea, and paroxysmal nocturnal dyspnea may occur, heralding the progression of left ventricular dysfunction. However, as discussed previously, mitral valve intervention to improve this volume overload can improve outcomes if performed promptly at the onset of symptoms.[16–18]

Echocardiography is the gold standard for diagnostic evaluation in patients presenting with suspected mitral regurgitation.[20] Typically, the mitral regurgitation severity is evaluated with semi-quantitative measurements initially.[10] These semi-quantitative measures include vena contract width, proximal isovelocity surface area (PISA) radius, pulmonary vein pattern, and color Doppler area. When these semi-quantitative measures suggest more severe mitral regurgitation, especially when two to three specific criteria for severe mitral regurgitation are met, performing a detailed quantitative analysis is recommended.[10] Quantitative methods include calculation of regurgitant volume, regurgitant fraction, and EROA with the continuity equation or by PISA method. Additionally, three-dimensional (3D) echocardiography can be utilized to determine the vena contracta area utilizing multiplanar reconstruction (**Fig. 2**).[21]

In particular, for primary mitral regurgitation, the echocardiographic determination of the mechanism of regurgitation and valve morphology (specifically the exact leaflet location of prolapse or flail) allows for valuable data to utilize for determining which surgical or transcatheter procedure is feasible. Other qualities of the mitral valve should also be assessed with echocardiography including calcification of the annulus or leaflets and length of the leaflets. Additionally, left ventricular size and function are important measures as these measures predict outcomes and can help determine the timing of valvular intervention.[10]

In cases where echocardiography is felt to be unsatisfactory for the evaluation of mitral regurgitation, or when there is a discrepancy between mitral regurgitation severity and clinical assessment, cardiac magnetic resonance imaging (CMR) may allow for further evaluation.[10] CMR allows for a thorough interrogation of the mitral valve apparatus.[22] Additionally, CMR allows for mitral regurgitation quantification through calculation of stroke volume differences between the right and left ventricles, and differences in stroke volume between the mitral inflow and aortic valve to calculate regurgitant volumes using phase-contrast imaging.[10,23] Severe mitral regurgitation as defined by CMR has also recently been noted as an independent predictor of post-mitral valve intervention improvement in left ventricular remodeling.[24]

MEDICAL THERAPY

Medical therapy for symptomatic mitral regurgitation is founded primarily on heart failure with reduced ejection fraction literature.[20,25] Specific evidence for therapy with angiotensin-converting enzyme (ACE) inhibitors, beta blockers, and aldosterone antagonists in mitral regurgitation populations is limited. Only small, randomized studies evaluating ACE inhibitors for the treatment of chronic, asymptomatic primary MR showed little evidence of benefit.[26,27] With respect to beta blockers, retrospective studies have shown a possible association between decreased mortality in patients with severe mitral regurgitation and normal left ventricular function.[28] Although vasodilators have a role in acute mitral regurgitation for afterload reduction, there is no literature to support the use of vasodilators for asymptomatic, normotensive patients with chronic primary mitral regurgitation. Overall, primary mitral regurgitation is managed with valve intervention, and there is only a narrow role for medical therapy in patients who would already require medical therapy for heart failure or hypertension.[20,25]

SURGICAL TREATMENT

The most well-studied and proven treatment of primary mitral regurgitation is surgical intervention. In general, mitral valve repair is preferable to mitral valve replacement. Repair of the mitral valve for primary mitral regurgitation can be accomplished through leaflet resection, plication, neochordae insertion, and chord transposition accompanied by an annuloplasty ring.[3,5,6] Mitral valve repair can be achieved with minimal operative mortality and outstanding long-term outcomes in properly selected patients.[3,5,6] The most recent literature suggests less than 1% for most patients.[29] Repair is preferable to replacement due to the lower operative mortality, superior long-term survival, and improved left ventricular function demonstrated

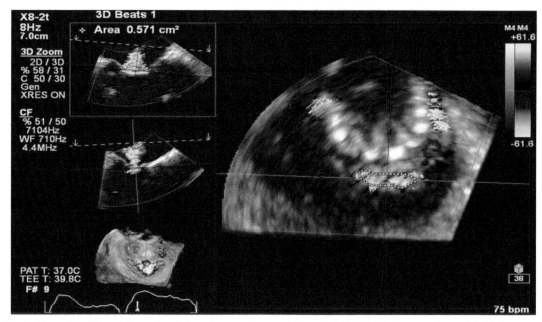

Fig. 2. Example of three-dimensional Doppler vena contracta area using multiplanar reconstruction. Reconstruction planes are aligned at the height of the two-dimensional vena contracta during systole in two different planes. The vena contracta area measures 0.571 cm² in this case, consistent with severe mitral regurgitation.

with mitral valve repair.[30] This survival benefit in repair compared to replacement is demonstrated for both posterior and bileaflet mitral valve prolapse but not in isolated anterior leaflet prolapse.[30] Accordingly, the risk of reoperation increases in patients with isolated anterior prolapse who undergo repair (1.6% per year) compared to those with isolated posterior repair (0.5% per year), bileaflet repair (0.9% per year), and mechanical valve replacement (0.66% per year).[30]

TRANSCATHETER INTERVENTION

Surgical evaluation for patients with moderate to severe or severe mitral regurgitation should include an assessment of operative risk. Patients with prohibitive mitral surgical risk (those with a 30-day Society of Thoracic Surgeons [STS]—predicted operative mortality of ≥ 8%) should be considered for transcatheter procedures.[31]

Transcatheter mitral valve procedures can be grouped into repair and replacement options. However, for primary mitral regurgitation, the only Food and Drug Administration (FDA)-approved options include edge-to-edge repair with MitraClip (Abbott Vascular, Santa Clara, CA) or PASCAL (Edwards Lifesciences; Irvine, CA).[31,32] Both devices produce edge-to-edge repair akin to the Alfieri stitch.[31,32]

The PASCAL device was recently FDA-approved based on a published head-to-head comparison

study of PASCAL and MitraClip which established the safety and effectiveness of the PASCAL system in meeting non-inferiority endpoints.[33] However, the most evaluated transcatheter mitral valve repair system is the MitraClip. The momentous trial for the MitraClip in treating primary mitral regurgitation was the EVEREST II trial. This trial randomized a majority (73%) of patients with primary mitral regurgitation to mitral valve repair or MitraClip with results showing no difference in survival, degree of improvement in left ventricular measurements, and functional capacity for MitraClip compared to surgery.[34] These results lead to the FDA approval of the MitraClip system for the management of primary mitral regurgitation.

Real-world data from nearly 3000 patients from the Society of Thoracic Surgery/American College of Cardiology Transcatheter Valve Therapy Registry receiving MitraClip intervention primarily for the indication of primary mitral regurgitation have confirmed the short-term safety (post-operative bleeding, stroke, device-related adverse events <2%) and efficacy of the MitraClip intervention.[35,36] Notably, the median mean gradient post-MitraClip intervention in these real world studies is 4 mm Hg.[35] Despite short-term efficacy and safety, long-term mortality remains substantial (25.8% mortality at 1 year), and heart failure morbidity persists (20.2% rehospitalization for heart failure at 1 year), although to a lesser degree than untreated primary mitral regurgitation.[35]

More contemporary data have shown that 30-day and 1-year outcomes for transcatheter edge-to-edge repair are improving as time and experience with these procedures continue to develop.[36] Of note, the introduction of transcatheter mitral repair has not significantly changed the overall surgical mitral valve repair volume but has led to fewer high-risk surgical operations and improved mortality within institutions adopting transcatheter therapy.[37]

Favorable anatomy for edge-to-edge repair includes planimetered mitral valve area $\geq$ 4.0 cm^2, minimal grasping area calcification, coaptation length greater than 2 mm, coaptation depth less than 11 mm, flail gap less than 10 mm, and a flail width less than 15 mm.[34] However, recent literature has established that advancements since mitral valve edge-to-edge intervention was initially introduced have allowed high transcatheter procedural success even in those with complex mitral valve anatomy, particularly with the PASCAL device.[38] Although these transcatheter repair devices are currently only approved for symptomatic patients with primary mitral regurgitation with favorable anatomy, and prohibitive surgical risk, there are ongoing trials evaluating these devices in patients with moderate and low surgical risks.

TIMING OF INTERVENTION

The rationale for the appropriate timing of mitral valve intervention with respect to primary mitral regurgitation is based largely on evaluating outcomes from natural history studies compared to studies of surgical intervention. These studies have shown improved outcomes with surgery performed for symptomatic primary mitral regurgitation.[39] Specifically, patients with severe chronic primary mitral regurgitation without surgical intervention have an estimated annual mortality rate of 6% and an annual cardiac event rate of 10%.[39] By comparison, immediate mortality post-mitral valve repair surgery varies from 1% to 2% for patients aged 75 years or younger.[39] Incidence of sudden death is similarly reduced when surgery is performed for flail mitral leaflet compared to no intervention.[17] However, improved outcomes with surgery rely on selecting patients with low surgical risk and referral to surgical centers of excellence. Other additional factors that portend to worse outcomes with medical therapy alone and may justify earlier mitral valve intervention are discussed below and include symptom onset, left ventricular function and size, atrial fibrillation, and pulmonary hypertension (**Fig. 3**).

Symptom Onset

Intervention promptly at symptom onset is one of the most important factors when considering when to intervene in patients with severe primary mitral regurgitation. Intervening early when patients are only minimally symptomatic has been shown to improve outcomes. This was demonstrated in multiple studies that retrospectively evaluated outcomes in patients with severe primary mitral regurgitation with both mild and more advanced symptoms.[40,41] These studies revealed that those patients with more severe symptoms (NYHA class III/IV) have significantly higher mortality compared to those with fewer symptoms (NYHA class II). However, worse outcomes have been demonstrated even with mild symptoms, and thus, even asymptomatic patients may benefit from early mitral valve intervention, especially in the presence of other factors that portend worse outcomes such as left ventricular dysfunction.[40]

Left Ventricular Size and Function

Pre-intervention left ventricular function is an important predictor of outcomes with primary mitral regurgitation intervention. A retrospective study of echocardiographic predictors of outcomes in primary mitral regurgitation intervention demonstrated that survival precipitously dropped when the LVEF dropped below 60%.[42] Similarly, in patients with flail leaflet, the presence of left ventricular dysfunction increased the risk of sudden death.[16] Additionally, pre-intervention left ventricular end-systolic diameter greater than 40 mm has been shown to foretell persistent left ventricular dilatation and dysfunction.[20,25,43]

Atrial Fibrillation and Pulmonary Hypertension

In addition to symptom burden and left ventricular function, the presence of atrial fibrillation and pulmonary hypertension (pulmonary artery systolic pressure $\geq$ 55 mm Hg) have been associated with worse outcomes in severe primary mitral regurgitation and are considered indications for intervention even in the asymptomatic patient. Both atrial fibrillation (by way of continued atrial remodeling) and pulmonary hypertension (by way of continued LV volume overload leading to post-capillary elevations in pulmonary pressures) would be expected to progressively worsen without mitral valve intervention. This progression in combination with worsened outcomes in previous studies is the rationale for using these markers as indications for severe primary mitral regurgitation intervention even in the absence of symptoms.[44–46]

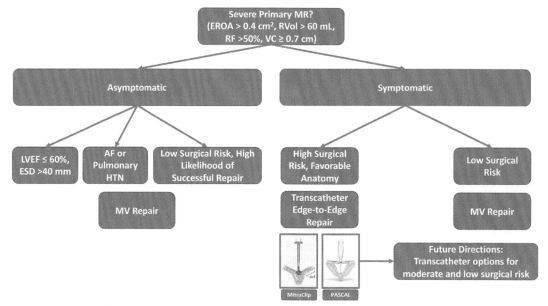

Fig. 3. The first step in evaluation of primary mitral regurgitation requires determination of severity with echocardiography. Once the primary mitral regurgitation is determined to be severe, determination of timing of intervention depends on presence of symptoms, left ventricular dimensions and function, and surgical risk. Other factors that would favor intervention include presence of atrial fibrillation or pulmonary hypertension. Candidates for intervention need to be further stratified into those best suited for surgery or transcatheter intervention. Future directions for severe primary mitral regurgitation likely will include multiple options for transcatheter interventions (outside MitraClip and PASCAL) and may include those patients at moderate or low surgical risk. AF, atrial fibrillation; EROA, effective regurgitant orifice area; ESD, end-systolic diameter; HTN, hypertension; LVEF, left ventricular ejection fraction; MR, mitral regurgitation; MV, mitral valve; RF, regurgitant fraction; RVol, regurgitant volume; VC, vena contracta. (*Data from* Otto CM, Nishimura RA, Bonow RO, et al. 2020 ACC/AHA Guideline for the Management of Patients With Valvular Heart Disease: Executive Summary: A Report of the American College of Cardiology/American Heart Association Joint Committee on Clinical Practice Guidelines [published correction appears in Circulation. 2021 Feb 2;143(5):e228] [published correction appears in Circulation. 2021 Mar 9;143(10):e784]. *Circulation.* 2021;143(5):e35-e71. MitraClip is a trademark of Abbott or its related companies. Reproduced with permission of Abbott, © 2022. All rights reserved. *Courtesy of* Edwards Lifescience, Chicago, IL.)

THE GROWING BURDEN AND UNDERTREATMENT OF MITRAL REGURGITATION

Over 30,000 mitral valve surgeries are performed each year, with most of these surgeries being performed for the indication of mitral regurgitation.[7] It is estimated that 1.3 million US adults suffer from isolated mitral regurgitation with a projected prevalence of 2.3 million by 2030.[47] Despite evidence of a growing burden of mitral regurgitation, patients were historically denied surgery due to advanced age, impaired LVEF, and comorbidity. However, these data may reflect patients referred too late in the disease process at a time before widely available transcatheter options for higher-risk patients.[48] A group at the Mayo Clinic in Olmsted County, MN, retrospectively reviewed 1294 patients diagnosed with moderate or severe mitral regurgitation and found that all subgroups of these patients (including those without symptoms and with normal left ventricular function and measurements) had increased risk of mortality and adverse cardiac outcomes (including 76% who ultimately developed heart failure) over a median follow-up of approximately 5 years.[49] Despite these worsening outcomes, only a small percentage overall (15%) of patients underwent mitral valve surgery. Even those with favorable anatomy for surgery, low comorbidities, and normal ejection had a low percentage of referral for surgery.[49] The excess mortality and high prevalence of heart failure in untreated mitral regurgitation illuminate the need for further developments in mitral valve intervention. Reassuringly, studies to remedy this situation are underway with potentially more patients becoming eligible for treatment with the continued development and approval of less invasive strategies beyond the MitraClip and PASCAL devices. This will be especially true if these therapies are approved for those patients at moderate and low surgical risk, for which studies are currently underway.

SUMMARY

Mitral valve disease, especially mitral regurgitation, is a frequent etiology of congestive heart failure. Primary mitral regurgitation is best treated with intervention as soon as symptoms arise or if there is concomitant left ventricular dysfunction, pulmonary hypertension, or atrial fibrillation. Surgical intervention improves outcomes in low-surgical-risk patients, compared to those managed medically. For those at high surgical risk, transcatheter options provide less invasive repair and replacement interventions while providing comparable outcomes to surgery. However, even those patients with few comorbidities and normal left ventricular parameters exhibit excess mortality and adverse outcomes with a high percentage developing heart failure if their primary mitral regurgitation is not intervened upon. Despite this excess of adverse outcomes, mitral valve intervention is infrequent. The excess mortality and high prevalence of heart failure in untreated mitral regurgitation illuminate the need for further developments in mitral valve intervention. This need will ideally be fulfilled by developing less invasive percutaneous interventions beyond MitraClip and PASCAL and expanding eligibility to these procedures beyond only those at high surgical risk.

CLINICS CARE POINTS

- Echocardiography is the gold standard for diagnosis of primary mitral regurgitation
- Patients with severe primary mitral regurgitation should be evaluated for heart failure symptoms, atrial fibrillation, pulmonary hypertension, and evidence of reduced LVEF and dilated left ventricular dimensions evaluation as these factors predict worse outcomes and guide the timing of intervention
- Severe primary mitral regurgitation is treated with surgical or transcatheter intervention as no specific medical therapy has proven beneficial in these patients
- Evaluation of surgical risk is key in deciding surgical versus transcatheter approaches to mitral valve intervention for severe primary mitral regurgitation
- Early surgical or transcatheter mitral valve intervention can improve outcomes substantially

FUNDING

This research did not receive any specific grant from funding agencies in the public, commercial, or not-for-profit sectors.

DISCLOSURES

None.

REFERENCES

1. Nkomo VT, Gardin JM, Skelton TN, et al. Burden of valvular heart diseases: a population-based study. Lancet 2006;368(9540):1005–11.
2. Silbiger JJ. Anatomy, mechanics, and pathophysiology of the mitral annulus. Am Heart J 2012; 164(2):163–76.
3. Enriquez-Sarano M, Avierinos JF, Messika-Zeitoun D, et al. Quantitative determinants of the outcome of asymptomatic mitral regurgitation. N Engl J Med 2005;352(9):875–83.
4. Mauri L, Foster E, Glower DD, et al. 4-year results of a randomized controlled trial of percutaneous repair versus surgery for mitral regurgitation. J Am Coll Cardiol 2013;62(4):317–28.
5. Mohty D, Orszulak TA, Schaff HV, et al. Very long-term survival and durability of mitral valve repair for mitral valve prolapse. Circulation 2001;104(12 Suppl 1):I1–7.
6. Suri RM, Vanoverschelde JL, Grigioni F, et al. Association between early surgical intervention vs watchful waiting and outcomes for mitral regurgitation due to flail mitral valve leaflets. JAMA 2013;310(6): 609–16.
7. Bowdish ME, D'Agostino RS, Thourani VH, et al. STS Adult Cardiac Surgery Database: 2021 Update on Outcomes, Quality, and Research. Ann Thorac Surg 2021;111(6):1770–80.
8. Anyanwu AC, Adams DH. Etiologic classification of degenerative mitral valve disease: Barlow's disease and fibroelastic deficiency. Semin Thorac Cardiovasc Surg 2007;19(2):90–6.
9. Adams DH, Rosenhek R, Falk V. Degenerative mitral valve regurgitation: best practice revolution. Eur Heart J 2010;31(16):1958–66.
10. Zoghbi WA, Adams D, Bonow RO, et al. Recommendations for Noninvasive Evaluation of Native Valvular Regurgitation: A Report from the American Society of Echocardiography Developed in Collaboration with the Society for Cardiovascular Magnetic Resonance. J Am Soc Echocardiogr 2017;30(4):303–71.
11. Avierinos JF, Gersh BJ, Melton LJ 3rd, et al. Natural history of asymptomatic mitral valve prolapse in the community. Circulation 2002;106(11):1355–61.
12. Kim S, Kuroda T, Nishinaga M, et al. Relationship between severity of mitral regurgitation and prognosis

of mitral valve prolapse: echocardiographic follow-up study. Am Heart J 1996;132(2 Pt 1):348–55.

13. Topilsky Y, Michelena H, Bichara V, et al. Mitral valve prolapse with mid-late systolic mitral regurgitation: pitfalls of evaluation and clinical outcome compared with holosystolic regurgitation. Circulation 2012; 125(13):1643–51.

14. Essayagh B, Sabbag A, Antoine C, et al. The Mitral Annular Disjunction of Mitral Valve Prolapse: Presentation and Outcome. JACC Cardiovasc Imaging 2021;14(11):2073–87.

15. Enriquez-Sarano M, Basmadjian AJ, Rossi A, et al. Progression of mitral regurgitation: a prospective Doppler echocardiographic study. J Am Coll Cardiol 1999;34(4):1137–44.

16. Rosenhek R, Rader F, Klaar U, et al. Outcome of watchful waiting in asymptomatic severe mitral regurgitation. Circulation 2006;113(18):2238–44.

17. Grigioni F, Tribouilloy C, Avierinos JF, et al. Outcomes in mitral regurgitation due to flail leaflets a multicenter European study. JACC Cardiovasc Imaging 2008;1(2):133–41.

18. Ling LH, Enriquez-Sarano M, Seward JB, et al. Early surgery in patients with mitral regurgitation due to flail leaflets: a long-term outcome study. Circulation 1997;96(6):1819–25.

19. El Sabbagh A, Reddy YNV, Nishimura RA. Mitral Valve Regurgitation in the Contemporary Era: Insights Into Diagnosis, Management, and Future Directions. JACC Cardiovasc Imaging 2018;11(4): 628–43.

20. Writing Committee M, Otto CM, Nishimura RA, et al. 2020 ACC/AHA Guideline for the Management of Patients With Valvular Heart Disease: Executive Summary: A Report of the American College of Cardiology/American Heart Association Joint Committee on Clinical Practice Guidelines. J Am Coll Cardiol 2021;77(4):450–500.

21. Zeng X, Levine RA, Hua L, et al. Diagnostic value of vena contracta area in the quantification of mitral regurgitation severity by color Doppler 3D echocardiography. Circ Cardiovasc Imaging 2011;4(5):506–13.

22. Buchner S, Poschenrieder F, Hamer OW, et al. Direct visualization of regurgitant orifice by CMR reveals differential asymmetry according to etiology of mitral regurgitation. JACC Cardiovasc Imaging 2011; 4(10):1088–96.

23. Kramer CM, Barkhausen J, Flamm SD, et al. Society for Cardiovascular Magnetic Resonance Board of Trustees Task Force on Standardized P. Standardized cardiovascular magnetic resonance (CMR) protocols 2013 update. J Cardiovasc Magn Reson 2013;15:91.

24. Uretsky S, Animashaun IB, Sakul S, et al. American Society of Echocardiography Algorithm for Degenerative Mitral Regurgitation: Comparison With CMR. JACC Cardiovasc Imaging 2022;15(5):747–60.

25. Otto CM, Nishimura RA, Bonow RO, et al. 2020 ACC/AHA Guideline for the Management of Patients With Valvular Heart Disease: A Report of the American College of Cardiology/American Heart Association Joint Committee on Clinical Practice Guidelines. Circulation 2021;143(5):e72–227.

26. Marcotte F, Honos GN, Walling AD, et al. Effect of angiotensin-converting enzyme inhibitor therapy in mitral regurgitation with normal left ventricular function. Can J Cardiol 1997;13(5):479–85.

27. Wisenbaugh T, Sinovich V, Dullabh A, et al. Six month pilot study of captopril for mildly symptomatic, severe isolated mitral and isolated aortic regurgitation. J Heart Valve Dis 1994;3(2):197–204.

28. Varadarajan P, Joshi N, Appel D, et al. Effect of Beta-blocker therapy on survival in patients with severe mitral regurgitation and normal left ventricular ejection fraction. Am J Cardiol 2008;102(5):611–5.

29. Badhwar V, Chikwe J, Gillinov AM, et al. Risk of Surgical Mitral Valve Repair for Primary Mitral Regurgitation. J Am Coll Cardiol 2023;81(7):636–48.

30. Suri RM, Schaff HV, Dearani JA, et al. Survival advantage and improved durability of mitral repair for leaflet prolapse subsets in the current era. Ann Thorac Surg 2006;82(3):819–26.

31. Lim DS, Reynolds MR, Feldman T, et al. Improved functional status and quality of life in prohibitive surgical risk patients with degenerative mitral regurgitation after transcatheter mitral valve repair. J Am Coll Cardiol 2014;64(2):182–92.

32. Maisano F, La Canna G, Colombo A, et al. The evolution from surgery to percutaneous mitral valve interventions: the role of the edge-to-edge technique. J Am Coll Cardiol 2011;58(21):2174–82.

33. Lim DS, Smith RL, Gillam LD, et al. Randomized Comparison of Transcatheter Edge-to-Edge Repair for Degenerative Mitral Regurgitation in Prohibitive Surgical Risk Patients. JACC Cardiovasc Interv 2022;15(24):2523–36.

34. Feldman T, Foster E, Glower DD, et al. Percutaneous repair or surgery for mitral regurgitation. N Engl J Med 2011;364(15):1395–406.

35. Sorajja P, Vemulapalli S, Feldman T, et al. Outcomes With Transcatheter Mitral Valve Repair in the United States: An STS/ACC TVT Registry Report. J Am Coll Cardiol 2017;70(19):2315–27.

36. Mack M, Carroll JD, Thourani V, et al. Transcatheter Mitral Valve Therapy in the United States: A Report From the STS-ACC TVT Registry. J Am Coll Cardiol 2021;78(23):2326–53.

37. Lowenstern AM, Vekstein AM, Grau-Sepulveda M, et al. Impact of Transcatheter Mitral Valve Repair Availability on Volume and Outcomes of Surgical Repair. J Am Coll Cardiol 2023;81(6):521–32.

38. Hausleiter J, Lim DS, Gillam LD, et al. Transcatheter Edge-to-Edge Repair in Patients With Anatomically

Complex Degenerative Mitral Regurgitation. J Am Coll Cardiol 2023;81(5):431–42.

39. Enriquez-Sarano M, Akins CW, Vahanian A. Mitral regurgitation. Lancet 2009;373(9672):1382–94.

40. Gillinov AM, Mihaljevic T, Blackstone EH, et al. Should patients with severe degenerative mitral regurgitation delay surgery until symptoms develop? Ann Thorac Surg 2010;90(2):481–8.

41. Tribouilloy CM, Enriquez-Sarano M, Schaff HV, et al. Impact of preoperative symptoms on survival after surgical correction of organic mitral regurgitation: rationale for optimizing surgical indications. Circulation 1999;99(3):400–5.

42. Enriquez-Sarano M, Tajik AJ, Schaff HV, et al. Echocardiographic prediction of survival after surgical correction of organic mitral regurgitation. Circulation 1994;90(2):830–7.

43. Song JM, Kang SH, Lee EJ, et al. Echocardiographic predictors of left ventricular function and clinical outcomes after successful mitral valve repair: conventional two-dimensional versus speckle-tracking parameters. Ann Thorac Surg 2011;91(6):1816–23.

44. Grigioni F, Benfari G, Vanoverschelde JL, et al. Long-Term Implications of Atrial Fibrillation in Patients With Degenerative Mitral Regurgitation. J Am Coll Cardiol 2019;73(3):264–74.

45. Szymanski C, Magne J, Fournier A, et al. Usefulness of preoperative atrial fibrillation to predict outcome and left ventricular dysfunction after valve repair for mitral valve prolapse. Am J Cardiol 2015; 115(10):1448–53.

46. Vahanian A, Beyersdorf F, Praz F, et al. 2021 ESC/EACTS Guidelines for the management of valvular heart disease. Eur J Cardio Thorac Surg 2021; 60(4):727–800.

47. d'Arcy JL, Coffey S, Loudon MA, et al. Large-scale community echocardiographic screening reveals a major burden of undiagnosed valvular heart disease in older people: the OxVALVE Population Cohort Study. Eur Heart J 2016;37(47):3515–22.

48. Mirabel M, Iung B, Baron G, et al. What are the characteristics of patients with severe, symptomatic, mitral regurgitation who are denied surgery? Eur Heart J 2007;28(11):1358–65.

49. Dziadzko V, Clavel MA, Dziadzko M, et al. Outcome and undertreatment of mitral regurgitation: a community cohort study. Lancet 2018;391(10124): 960–9.

Secondary Mitral Regurgitation and Heart Failure
Current Advances in Diagnosis and Management

Muhammed Gerçek, MD[a,b,*], Akhil Narang, MD[b],
Jyothy J. Puthumana, MD[b], Charles J. Davidson, MD[b], Volker Rudolph, MD[a]

KEYWORDS

- Secondary mitral regurgitation • Transcatheter mitral valve repair • MitraClip • PASCAL
- Transcatheter mitral valve replacement

KEY POINTS

- Secondary mitral regurgitation (SMR) still remains a challenging disease and requires a multiparametric approach in imaging and diagnostic tools and a multidisciplinary heart team to individualize the treatment strategy for each patient.
- Guideline-directed medical therapy remains the cornerstone of all treatment approaches of SMR.
- Transcatheter edge-to-edge repair (TEER) first intervention to have an impact on prognosis in this patient cohort, if the COAPT criteria are met.
- Through the expansion of transcatheter therapy options with new "edge-to-edge" systems and newer transcatheter mitral valve replacement strategies (TMVR), several new treatment options will be soon available that will enable individualized therapy in these challenging patients.
- Nevertheless, these new TMVR systems have to prove noninferiority against the already established TEER technologies.

INTRODUCTION: MITRAL REGURGITATION PATHOPHYSIOLOGY AND PROGNOSIS

Mitral regurgitation (MR) is the most common valvular lesion in the western world and is associated with significant mortality and morbidity.[1] The overall prevalence of clinically significant MR is ~2% with an increase associated with increasing age and observed in about 10% of patients aged 75 years or older.[2] Additionally, the prevalence of MR is still expected to increase further due to the society aging globally but even more so in the west. To date, more than 2 million Americans are

suffering from significant MR.[1] Generally, MR is caused by primary (degenerative) and secondary (functional) pathologic conditions. Primary MR (PMR) is caused by structural abnormalities of the mitral valve and the mitral valve apparatus including papillary muscles and chordae while the underlying cause of secondary MR (SMR) is multifactorial.[3] Morphologic changes in the left ventricular (LV) geometry lead to ventricular and mitral annular dilation with restriction of the mitral valve leaflets resulting in insufficient coaptation of the normal or almost normal mitral leaflets due to, for example, fibrosis or stiffening of the

a Clinic for General and Interventional Cardiology/Angiology, Heart- und Diabetes Center NRW, Ruhr University Bochum, Bad Oeynhausen, Germany; b Northwestern University, Feinberg School of Medicine, Chicago, IL, USA
* Corresponding author. Clinic for General and Interventional Cardiology/Angiology, Heart- und Diabetes Center NRW, Ruhr University Bochum, Georgstraße 11, Bad Oeynhausen 32545, Germany.
E-mail address: mugercek@hdz-nrw.de

Heart Failure Clin 19 (2023) 307–315
https://doi.org/10.1016/j.hfc.2023.02.010
1551-7136/23/© 2023 Elsevier Inc. All rights reserved.

papillary muscles, in many cases following myocardial infarction.[4] In the past decade, atrial functional MR with left atrial enlargement has been recognized as an important entity of functional MR: Atrial FMR is mechanistically linked to annular enlargement, dysfunctional annular contraction, and atrial-caused leaflet tethering commonly described in patients with atrial fibrillation and heart failure with preserved ejection fraction.[5]

If left untreated, the prognosis of acute severe MR is generally very poor.[6] Acute MR caused by papillary muscle or chordal rupture results in acute pulmonary edema and cardiogenic shock with extremely poor prognosis without emergency cardiac surgery.[6] In chronic SMR, the malcoaptation of the leaflets with associated large resultant regurgitant volumes (RVs) can be compensated by the LV for some time and hence patients with chronic MR may remain asymptomatic for a long time.[7] With progression of disease, patients present with dyspnea and limited functional status related to increased pulmonary capillary pressures and poor forward stroke volume.[7] Chronic SMR is associated with significantly poor 5-year outcomes of cardiac death, hospitalization due to heart failure and new-onset of atrial fibrillation.[8] Development of pulmonary hypertension, ventricular dilation and dysfunction, atrial dilatation, and atrial fibrillation have been shown to be predictors for worse outcomes.[6] Therefore, early and appropriate diagnosis, triage, and management of SMR are of critical importance and contemporary evidence in SMR supporting this will be summarized in this review.

DIAGNOSTICS IN MITRAL REGURGITATION

Grading the severity of MR in SMR can be very challenging as abnormal findings of left atrial enlargement, abnormal pulmonary venous flow, and so forth could be caused by the underlying LV pathologic condition itself rather than the MR.[9]

Comprehensive echocardiography including volumetric measurements, 2D and color Doppler imaging, 3D imaging, and strain imaging continues to be the cornerstone and the initial study of choice to assess SMR.[10] A multiparametric approach to assess MR including qualitative assessment (Mitra valve morphology, color flow jet area, flow convergence, continuous Doppler jet), semiquantitative (Vena contracta, pulmonary vein flow, mitral inflow, mitral time-velocity integral to aortic time-velocity integral-ratio), quantitative (effective regurgitation orifice area, RV, regurgitant fraction), and morphologic accurate chamber measurements to document left atrial and

ventricular enlargement is warranted (**Box 1**).[11] Not surprisingly, there have been disparities in the past with regard to the cutoff values for defining severe SMR, and also between the European and the American Guidelines.[12,13] However, the 2021 European guidelines for the management of valvular heart disease align with recommendations of the American Society of Echocardiography valvular regurgitation guidelines from 2017 for comprehensive evaluation and quantification of SMR.[3,10,11]

Accurate and reproducible quantification of LV volumes and MR seems to be crucial for the prediction of outcomes and adoption of management strategies as suggested by guidelines.[8] The most

---

Box 1
Severe functional mitral regurgitation criteria based on two-dimensional echocardiography

Parameter	Criteria for Severe Secondary MR
Qualitative	
Mitral valve morphology	Normal leaflets but with severe tethering, poor leaflet coaptation (sometimes with minor leaflet thickening and annular calcification)
Color flow jet area	Large central jet (>50% of the left atrium) or eccentric wall impinging jet of variable size
Flow convergence	Large throughout systole
Continuous Doppler jet	Holosystolic/dense/triangular
Semiquantitative	
Vena contracta width	≥ 7 (≥ 8 mm for biplane)
Pulmonary vein flow	Systolic flow reversal
Mitral inflow	E-wave dominant (>1.2 m/s)
Quantitative	
Effective regurgitation orifice area	≥ 40 mm^2 (may be ≥ 30 mm^2 if elliptical regurgitant orifice area)
Regurgitant volume	≥ 60 mL (may be ≥ 45 mL in low-flow conditions)
Regurgitant fraction	$\geq 50\%$
Structural	Dilated left ventricle and/or atrium

Data from Refs.[3,10,11]

important sources of error are underestimation of absolute LV volumes based on 2-dimensional echocardiography and underestimation of SMR based on proximal isovelocity surface area (PISA)—derived from effective regurgitation orifice area (EROA) and MR-RV.[14] The PISA method is prone to underestimate EROA and MR-RV severity compared with results of cardiac magnetic resonance (CMR) or 3-dimensional echocardiography especially in SMR in which the orifice geometry is noncircular and MR changes dynamically over the systolic time interval and strongly dependent on loading conditions.

Considered together, there has been a general agreement that regurgitant fraction greater than 50% may be the best measure of severe MR.[14–16] Yet regurgitant fraction may be difficult to calculate with 2-dimensional echocardiography and was not universally available even in the randomized controlled trials. More accurate and reproducible approaches to quantifying MR—such as 3-dimensional echocardiography and CMR may become the reference standard for MR quantification and will be important to be studied in future trials.[17]

TREATMENT OF SECONDARY MITRAL REGURGITATION
Medical Therapy

In patients with heart failure with reduced ejection fraction, guideline-directed medical therapy (GDMT) is the first-line therapeutic approach as recommended in the European as well as American guidelines (**Fig. 1**). Treatment with beta-blockers, renin–angiotensin–aldosterone system antagonists,[3,10] and most recently angiotensin receptor neprilysin inhibitor (ARNI) and sodium glucose transporter 2 (SGLT2) inhibitor therapy may result in LV unloading, reverse remodeling, and pleiotropic drug effects secondarily reducing SMR.[18,19] ARNI and SGLT2 therapy were not part of GDMT during recently published randomized clinical trials in SMR and heart failure and hence additional benefits for reduction of MR with the use of these agents have not been systematically studied. Additionally, indications for cardiac resynchronization therapy should be evaluated and if symptoms persist despite optimization of GDMT, mitral valve procedures should be considered and performed before further deterioration of LV function and enlargement.[10] However, all patients with SMR should be reviewed by the Heart Team that includes an imaging expert, an experienced interventional cardiologist, a cardiac surgeon with an expertise in mitral valve surgery, and a heart failure specialist.

Surgical Therapy

Despite the association of SMR with mortality, there is no convincing evidence that surgical correction of SMR is superior to medical therapy.[20,21] Yet, guidelines based on data from the STICH trial recommend that mitral valve repair should be considered in patients with significant SMR undergoing concomitant coronary artery bypass grafting (class IIA).[10,22]

Inconsistencies exist with regard to the optimal surgical treatment strategy with regard to mitral valve replacement versus repair. In a randomized controlled study, there was no difference in mortality between repair and replacement but a higher rate of recurrent MR in the repair-group at 2 years.[23] However, Girdauskas and colleagues suggest that all patients with SMR need individualized evaluation of the pathologic condition because patients with atrial MR with predominant left atrial dilation, mitral annular dilation with flattening of the annulus, and central malcoaptation of the leaflets may benefit from mitral valve repair, whereas patients with predominant LV dilation and leaflet tethering into the LV cavity might benefit more from a replacement strategy because the disease progression with continued remodeling and enlargement of the left ventricle could result in recurrent MR after repair when compared with replacement.[24]

The ongoing MATTERHORN study (NCT02371512), which randomized patients with SMR to TEER or surgical mitral valve therapy will further help to guide decision-making for these patients in the future. Results of this study are expected in 2024.

Interventional Therapy

Transcatheter edge-to-edge repair (TEER) using the MitraClip system (Abbott Vascular, Santa Clara, CA) was approved in 2008 in Europe. Between 2014 and 2020, there was a 10-fold increase in transcatheter mitral valve procedures in Europe, mostly among patients with SMR.[25] However, until 2018, results in patients with SMR from randomized clinical trials compared with GDMT were lacking. In 2018, results of 2 randomized trials, the COAPT trial and MITRA FR trial, comparing TEER with the MitraClip system and GDMT versus GDMT alone were published, which added further fuel to the controversies about the role and timing of TEER among SMR patients with heart failure.[26,27] Both studies included patients with LV systolic dysfunction (COAPT 20%–50%, MITRA-FR 15%–40%) and SMR. Severe MR was graded in MITRA FR as EROA greater than 20 mm^2, MR-RV of 30 mL, whereas in COAPT, severe MR was defined as EROA greater than

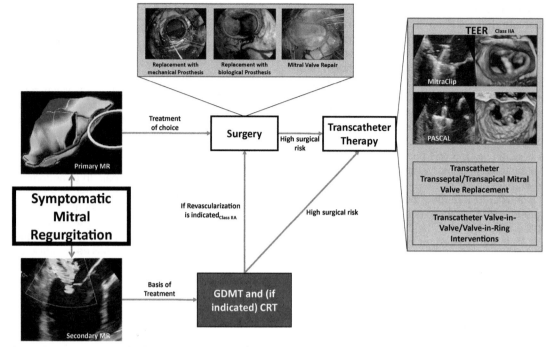

Fig. 1. Treatment strategies in symptomatic mitral regurgitation.

30 mm^2 and MR-RV greater than 30 mL. Additionally, patients with severe tricuspid regurgitation (TR) and severe pulmonary hypertension were excluded from the COAPT study.

tAt 2-year follow-up, the COAPT study showed a remarkable 50% reduction of hospitalization (Number needed to treat 3.1, 95%CI [1.9–7.9]; $P < .001$) due to heart failure and a 40% reduction in mortality (Number needed to treat 5.9, 95%CI [3.9–11.7]; $P < .001$) among patients who were randomized to the MitraClip procedure in addition to GDMT compared with patients with GDMT alone. These beneficial effects in the TEER arm remained stable at 3 years and also at 5 years of follow-up and patients who eventually crossed over to the TEER arm were noted to have a comparable benefit with this therapy compared with those originally assigned to the TEER arm along with GDMT.[28,29]

In contrast, 1-year and 2-years data from the MITRA-FR study showed no significant reduction of death or hospitalization.[27,30]

Several potential explanations for these drastically differing results have been discussed. One of the most important differences between both trials was that optimal GDMT was managed by a heart failure specialist and was confirmed by a central eligibility committee in COAPT, whereas the definition of GDMT was left to the discretion of the study site in MITRA-FR. In addition, in MITRA-FR changes in heart failure medication throughout the trial were not assessed.

Moreover, the differing inclusion criteria mentioned above, resulted in patients with less MR, and more dilated left ventricles in MITRA-FR, as indicated by a higher indexed left ventricular end-diastolic volume (LVEDVi). These differences were elaborated in the concept of disproportionate versus proportionate MR, which somewhat intuitively concludes that patients who have more MR and less remodeling (disproportionate MR) are more likely to respond to TEER, an intervention that directly reduces MR and only indirectly affects the left ventricle.[4] Packer and Grayburn proposed a cutoff of 0.14 for the ratio of EROA to LVEDV to separate proportionate from disproportionate MR (**Fig. 2**). They noted that there were more patients with proportionate MR in the MITRA-FR cohort and argued that this accounted for outcome differences. Their analysis of a small subgroup of patients in COAPT with proportionate MR (EROA of 30 cm^2 or less and LVEDVi >96 mL/m^2) experienced no significant effect of TEER on the outcome measures at 1 year, similar to the outcomes noted in MITRA-FR. All other subgroups with more MR and/or smaller LV end-diastolic volumes were determined to have disproportionate MR and benefited from TEER, as had been reported for the entire COAPT cohort. Lindenfeld and colleagues further explored these concepts by comparing the same MITRA-FR-like subset of the COAPT cohort (group 1, n = 56) with all other COAPT participants (group 2, n = 492).[31] They

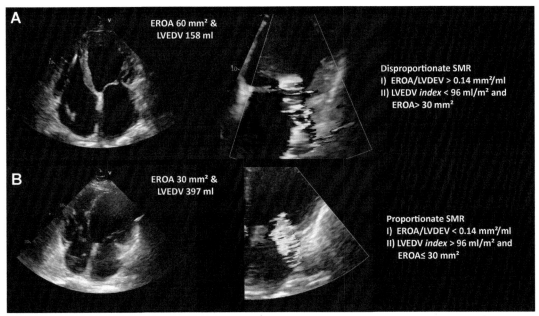

Fig. 2. Disproportionate and proportionate mitral regurgitation. Disproportionate MR defined as EROA/LVEDV ratio greater than 0.14 mm²/mL (I) or EROA ≤30 mm² and LVEDV index greater than 96 mL/m²) (II) (*A*) and proportionate MR (*B*) defined as EROA/LVEDV ratio ≤0.14 mm²/mL (I) or EROA ≤30 mm² and LVEDV index greater than 96 mL/m² (II).

extended a more granular analysis of groups, divided by LVEDVi (with the same cutoff of 96 mL/m²) and varying severities of MR, based on not only EROA but also MR-RV, and using American Society of Echocardiography recommended cut-offs for mild, moderate, and severe regurgitation. The latter was designed to retest the hypothesis that the disproportionate-proportionate MR framework explains the different trial results.

This concept, although pathophysiology intriguing has to be put in the context of further potentially relevant technical differences between both trials, among which the most important ones are (1) a less-efficient MR reduction in MITRA-FR and (2) the observation that 28% of the treatment arm in MITRA-FR did not receive a TEER.

Another important aspect is the treatment of concomitant secondary TR, which is common in patients with MR. Despite the lack of strong evidence and conclusive data, Sisinni and colleagues suggest that either isolated mitral TEER, a concomitant approach, and a watchful waiting strategy could be considered depending on the clinical and echocardiographic presentation of right ventricular function, pulmonary hypertension, and the phenotype of TR.[32]

Considered together, this discussion shows the complexity in SMR patient selection for TEER interventions. However, the results from the COAPT trial led to FDA approval in 2019 and led to a class

IIa indication for TEER intervention for SMR in the AHA/ACC guidelines for the management of patients with valvular heart disease when they present eligible anatomic criteria (COAPT criteria) and without a significantly dilated left ventricle (left ventricular end-systolic diameter [LVESD] ≤70 mm).[10]

Prediction Analysis in Patients with Secondary Mitral Regurgitation

At transcatheter valve therapies (TVT) 2022, updated data from the EXPAND registry showed that MitraClip treatment in SMR patients with non-COAPT-like anatomy (n = 160) was less effective, yet showed remarkable clinical improvement and similar 1-year outcomes compared with patients with COAPT-like anatomy (n = 125). The EXPAND registry also confirmed that a high proportion of patients with SMR were treated outside COAPT eligibility criteria, which makes further in-depth analysis of these patients and observations with longer duration of follow-up clearly warranted.

However, subgroup analysis of the COAPT study could identify important predictors for outcome, which could further inform patient selection. One important aspect in patient selection is the right heart. Hahn and colleagues showed in the COAPT cohort, that patients with significant

TR had worse clinical and echocardiographic characteristics and a worse clinical outcome compared with patients with mild TR.[33] Similar to that, Brener and colleagues showed that advanced right ventricular dysfunction assessed by the right ventricular-pulmonary artery coupling defined as right ventricular free wall longitudinal strain to pulmonary systolic artery pressure ratio under 0.5%/mm Hg was a strong predictor of worse outcomes during 2 years of follow-up in patients with SMR whether they remained on GDMT alone or underwent TEER.[34] Using these findings Shah and colleagues developed a risk prediction model for death and heart failure hospitalization utilizing 4 clinical (New York Heart Association class, chronic obstructive pulmonary disease, atrial fibrillation, and Chronic kidney disease) and 4 echocardiographic parameters (LV ejection fraction, LV end-diastolic diameter, right ventricular systolic pressure, and TR) in patients with SMR.[35] Additionally, Stolz and colleagues showed that classifying patients who underwent TEER procedures into heart failure with reduced ejection fraction and SMR according to extramitral cardiac involvement (stage 1: LV involvement; stage 2: left atrial involvement; stage 3: right ventricular involvement; stage 4: biventricular failure) may provide prognostic information in terms of survival and symptomatic improvement.[36]

Transcatheter Edge-to-Edge Repair Interventions in Patients with Advanced Heart Failure

Godino and colleagues studied a group of advanced heart failure patients with SMR from the MitraBridge Registry awaiting heart transplantation who underwent a TEER intervention were.[37] In total, 119 patients were included with severely impaired LV ejection fraction (26%). Procedural success was achieved in 87.5% of the patients and two-thirds of the patients remained free from adverse events (death, HF hospitalization, LV assist device implantation, heart transplantation) at 1 year and 23% no longer met indications for heart transplantation due to clinical improvement. This study suggested that TEER interventions can be safely performed as a bridge in advanced heart failure (HF) patients with SMR with high success rates and clinically important short-term clinical benefits.

Future Directions for Transcatheter Interventions in Secondary Mitral Regurgitation Patients

In 2019, another edge-to-edge System, the PASCAL System (Edwards, Irvine, CA) was approved in Europe, which is in the meantime available in 2 different sizes. This system provided for the first time a central spacer and independent leaflet clasping. With the introduction of the newest generation of the MitraClip system, providing different device sizes as well as now also independent leaflet grasping a broad spectrum of TEER devices are now available with increased safety, predictable results and the varied morphology of mitral valve pathologic condition that can be successfully treated. The early feasibility trial for the PASCAL device (CLASP study) showed a robust and safe MR reduction in primary as well as SMR at 30 days, 1 year, and 2 years. Sustained MR reduction (MR ≤ 1+ in 78% and MR ≤ 2 + 97%) in 124 patients (on average 75 years, 56% men, 69% SMR, 31% PMR) undergoing TEER with the PASCAL system and at 2 years, the survival rate was 80% with 85% reduction in annualized heart failure hospitalization.[38–40] First results in the CLASP IID trial randomizing patients with PMR 2:1 for the PASCAL or the MitraClip showed a non-inferiority of the PASCAL system against the MitraClip system, which resulted in FDA approval of the PASCAL system in September 2022 in patients with PMR.[41]

Real-world data from European centers performing propensity score matched analysis of PASCAL and MitraClip procedures (PMR and SMR) showed comparable acute (n = 604) and 1-year (n = 184) results with sustained MR reduction (MR ≤ 1+ in at least 70% of the patients at 1 year).[42–44] The pivotal CLASP IIF IDE trial is randomizing MitraClip to PASCAL and is currently enrolling.

TRANSCATHETER MITRAL VALVE REPLACEMENT

There are several transcatheter mitral valve replacements in pivotal or early feasibility trials.

In Europe, the transapical Tendyne system (Abbott Vascular, Santa Clara, CA) is already approved and is showing remarkable results. The initial feasibility study included 100 selected patients with primary and secondary MR with high-operative risk. The transapical procedure was performed with high safety and patients reported significant symptom relief and improvement in the 6-minute-walking test with a 1-year survival rate of 72%.[45,46] A 2-year follow-up data confirmed sustained MR reduction and a 2-year all-cause mortality of 39% with lower hospitalization rates in the second year.[47] Moreover, real-world data from 108 patients (43% female, mean age 75 ± 7 years, mean STS-PROM 7.2 ± 5.3%) treated with the Tendyne procedure showed high technical success rate (96%) with efficient and durable MR reduction (MR $\leq$ 1+ in all cases at follow up [n = 74]), which also translated to symptomatic improvement (73% in NYHA class I-II, P < .001).[48] The CHOICE Registry also showed that transcatheter mitral valve replacement (n = 229) with 10 different dedicated devices resulted in sustained MR elimination and functional improvement at 1 year in patients with SMR with large LV dimensions.[49] Although several transseptal mitral valve replacement devices are in trials, none is approved in the United States or Europe.

Mitral Valve-In-Valve and Valve-In-Ring Interventions

The number of patients with history of mitral valve surgery undergoing mitral valve-in-valve (MViV) or valve-in-ring-procedures (MViR) with transcatheter aortic valve replacement prosthesis in increasing every year.[25] Whisenant and colleagues reported that procedural success was achieved in 96.6% of 1500 high-risk patients who received the balloon-expandable Sapien 3 prosthesis (Edwards, Irvine, CA) and mortality was 16.7% at 1-year follow-up.[50] Simonato reported from the VIVID registry that patients with valve in ring procedure had a higher mortality and higher rate of relevant residual MR.[51] These findings were confirmed by Mack and colleagues who analyzed data received from the Society of Thoracic Surgeons/American College of Cardiology Transcatheter Valve Therapy Registry that patients with MViV had a lower mortality than patients with MViR at 30 days (4.7% vs 9.4%).[25]

One potential explanation is that MViR procedures with the current available transcatheter technologies are more challenging due to the anatomic subsets and the different construct of surgical rings that were implanted. Hence, proper case and device selection along with initial choice of surgical ring are even more important in this subgroup of patients to safely obtain the intended result.[25]

SUMMARY

SMR still remains a challenging disease and requires a multiparametric diagnostic approach as well as a multidisciplinary heart team to individualize the treatment strategy for each patient. GDMT remains the cornerstone of all treatment approaches of SMR. TEER is the first intervention to have an impact on prognosis in this patient cohort, if the COAPT criteria are met. If the COAPT criteria are not met in a patient with heart failure and significant SMR, the role of TEER interventions remains unclear although at least a symptomatic improvement could be expected. Through the expansion of transcatheter therapy options with new "edge-to-edge" systems and newer transcatheter mitral valve replacement strategies (TMVR), several new treatment options will be soon available that will enable individualized therapy in these challenging patients. Nevertheless, these new TMVR systems have to prove noninferiority and/or expansion of treatment options compared with the already established TEER technologies. The complexity of the mitral valve and its varied pathologic condition in patients with SMR with unmet need for individualization of transcatheter therapies will continue to keep the clinical and research tools in this arena very relevant for the near future.

CLINICS CARE POINTS

- Secondary mitral regurgitation (SMR) is a challenging disease and should be treated in centers with dedicated heart valve programs
- Grading the severity of SMR requires a multiparametric approach in imaging and diagnostic tools
- Guideline directed medical therapy remains the cornerstone of all treatment approaches of SMR
- Through the expansion of transcatheter therapy options with new "edge-to-edge" systems and newer transcatheter mitral valve replacement strategies a number of new treatment options will be soon available that will enable individualized therapy in these challenging patients.

DISCLOSURE

M. Gerçek has received research grants from the German Heart Foundation, Germany. J.J. Puthumana has received speaker Honoria from Abbott. C.J. Davidson received research grants from Abbott and Edwards, United State and is an uncompensated consultant for Edwards Lifesciences and consultant for Philips Healthcare. V. Rudolph has received research grants and speaker Honoria from Abbott and Edwards Lifesciences.

REFERENCES

1. Enriquez-Sarano M, Akins CW, Vahanian A. Mitral regurgitation. Lancet (London, England) 2009; 373(9672):1382–94.

2. Nkomo VT, Gardin JM, Skelton TN, et al. Burden of valvular heart diseases: a population-based study. Lancet (London, England) 2006;368(9540):1005–11.

3. Vahanian A, Beyersdorf F, Praz F, et al. 2021 ESC/EACTS Guidelines for the management of valvular heart disease: Developed by the Task Force for the management of valvular heart disease of the European Society of Cardiology (ESC) and the European Association for Cardio-Thoracic Surgery (EACTS). Eur Heart J 2021;43(7):561–632.

4. Grayburn PA, Sannino A, Packer M. Proportionate and Disproportionate Functional Mitral Regurgitation: A New Conceptual Framework That Reconciles the Results of the MITRA-FR and COAPT Trials. JACC Cardiovascular imaging 2019;12(2):353–62.

5. Farhan S, Silbiger JJ, Halperin JL, et al. Pathophysiology, Echocardiographic Diagnosis, and Treatment of Atrial Functional Mitral Regurgitation: JACC State-of-the-Art Review. J Am Coll Cardiol 2022;80(24):2314–30.

6. Barbieri A, Bursi F, Grigioni F, et al. Prognostic and therapeutic implications of pulmonary hypertension complicating degenerative mitral regurgitation due to flail leaflet: a multicenter long-term international study. Eur Heart J 2011;32(6):751–9.

7. Dziadzko V, Clavel MA, Dziadzko M, et al. Outcome and undertreatment of mitral regurgitation: a community cohort study. Lancet (London, England) 2018;391(10124):960–9.

8. Grigioni F, Avierinos JF, Ling LH, et al. Atrial fibrillation complicating the course of degenerative mitral regurgitation: determinants and long-term outcome. J Am Coll Cardiol 2002;40(1):84–92.

9. Grayburn PA, Thomas JD. Basic Principles of the Echocardiographic Evaluation of Mitral Regurgitation. JACC Cardiovascular imaging 2021;14(4):843–53.

10. Otto CM, Nishimura RA, Bonow RO, et al. ACC/AHA Guideline for the Management of Patients With Valvular Heart Disease: A Report of the American College of Cardiology/American Heart Association Joint Committee on Clinical Practice Guidelines. Circulation 2021;143(5):e35–71.

11. Zoghbi WA, Adams D, Bonow RO, et al. Recommendations for Noninvasive Evaluation of Native Valvular Regurgitation: A Report from the American Society of Echocardiography Developed in Collaboration with the Society for Cardiovascular Magnetic Resonance. J Am Soc Echocardiogr 2017;30(4):303–71.

12. Baumgartner H, Falk V, Bax JJ, et al. ESC/EACTS Guidelines for the management of valvular heart disease. Eur Heart J 2017;38(36):2739–91.

13. Nishimura RA, Otto CM, Bonow RO, et al. AHA/ACC Focused Update of the 2014 AHA/ACC Guideline for the Management of Patients With Valvular Heart Disease: A Report of the American College of Cardiology/American Heart Association Task Force on Clinical Practice Guidelines. Circulation 2017;135(25):e1159–95.

14. Hahn RT. Disproportionate Emphasis on Proportionate Mitral Regurgitation—Are There Better Measures of Regurgitant Severity? JAMA cardiology 2020;5(4):377–9.

15. Packer M, Grayburn PA. New evidence supporting a novel conceptual framework for distinguishing proportionate and disproportionate functional mitral regurgitation. JAMA cardiology 2020;5(4):469–75.

16. Gaasch WH, Aurigemma GP, Meyer TE. An appraisal of the association of clinical outcomes with the severity of regurgitant volume relative to end-diastolic volume in patients with secondary mitral regurgitation. JAMA cardiology 2020;5(4):476–81.

17. Uretsky S, Animashaun IB, Sakul S, et al. American Society of Echocardiography Algorithm for Degenerative Mitral Regurgitation: Comparison With CMR. JACC Cardiovascular imaging 2022;15(5):747–60.

18. Packer M, Anker SD, Butler J, et al. Cardiovascular and Renal Outcomes with Empagliflozin in Heart Failure. N Engl J Med 2020;383(15):1413–24.

19. Kang DH, Park SJ, Shin SH, et al. Angiotensin Receptor Neprilysin Inhibitor for Functional Mitral Regurgitation. Circulation 2019;139(11):1354–65.

20. Deja MA, Grayburn PA, Sun B, et al. Influence of mitral regurgitation repair on survival in the surgical treatment for ischemic heart failure trial. Circulation 2012;125(21):2639–48.

21. Acker MA, Parides MK, Perrault LP, et al. Mitral-valve repair versus replacement for severe ischemic mitral regurgitation. N Engl J Med 2014;370(1):23–32.

22. Tsang MYC, She L, Miller FA, et al. Differential Impact of Mitral Valve Repair on Outcome of Coronary Artery Bypass Grafting With or Without Surgical Ventricular Reconstruction in the Surgical Treatment for Ischemic Heart Failure (STICH) Trial. Struct Heart 2019;3(4):302–8.

23. Goldstein D, Moskowitz AJ, Gelijns AC, et al. Two-Year Outcomes of Surgical Treatment of Severe Ischemic Mitral Regurgitation. N Engl J Med 2016;374(4):344–53.

24. Girdauskas E, Pausch J, Harmel E, et al. Minimally invasive mitral valve repair for functional mitral regurgitation. Eur J Cardio Thorac Surg : official journal of the European Association for Cardio-thoracic Surgery 2019;55(Suppl 1):i17–25.

25. Mack M, Carroll JD, Thourani V, et al. Transcatheter Mitral Valve Therapy in the United States: A Report From the STS-ACC TVT Registry. J Am Coll Cardiol 2021;78(23):2326–53.

26. Stone GW, Lindenfeld J, Abraham WT, et al. Transcatheter Mitral-Valve Repair in Patients with Heart Failure. N Engl J Med 2018;379(24):2307–18.

27. Obadia JF, Messika-Zeitoun D, Leurent G, et al. Percutaneous Repair or Medical Treatment for

Secondary Mitral Regurgitation. N Engl J Med 2018; 379(24):2297–306.

28. Mack MJ, Lindenfeld J, Abraham WT, et al. 3-Year Outcomes of Transcatheter Mitral Valve Repair in Patients With Heart Failure. J Am Coll Cardiol 2021; 77(8):1029–40.

29. Stone GW, Abraham WT, Lindenfeld J, et al. COAPT Investigators. Five-Year Follow-up after Transcatheter Repair of Secondary Mitral Regurgitation. N Engl J Med 2023. https://doi.org/10.1056/NEJMoa2300213.

30. Iung B, Armoiry X, Vahanian A, et al. Percutaneous repair or medical treatment for secondary mitral regurgitation: outcomes at 2 years. Eur J Heart Fail 2019;21(12):1619–27.

31. Lindenfeld J, Abraham WT, Grayburn PA, et al. Association of Effective Regurgitation Orifice Area to Left Ventricular End-Diastolic Volume Ratio With Transcatheter Mitral Valve Repair Outcomes: A Secondary Analysis of the COAPT Trial. JAMA cardiology 2021;6(4):427–36.

32. Sisinni A, Taramasso M, Praz F, et al. Concomitant Transcatheter Edge-to-Edge Treatment of Secondary Tricuspid and Mitral Regurgitation: An Expert Opinion. JACC Cardiovasc Interv 2023;16(2): 127–39.

33. Hahn RT, Asch F, Weissman NJ, et al. Impact of Tricuspid Regurgitation on Clinical Outcomes: The COAPT Trial. J Am Coll Cardiol 2020;76(11): 1305–14.

34. Brener MI, Grayburn P, Lindenfeld J, et al. Right Ventricular–Pulmonary Arterial Coupling in Patients With HF Secondary MR. JACC Cardiovasc Interv 2021;14(20):2231–42.

35. Shah N, Madhavan MV, Gray WA, et al. Prediction of Death or HF Hospitalization in Patients With Severe FMR: The COAPT Risk Score. JACC Cardiovasc Interv 2022;15(19):1893–905.

36. Stolz L, Doldi PM, Orban M, et al. Staging Heart Failure Patients With Secondary Mitral Regurgitation Undergoing Transcatheter Edge-to-Edge Repair. JACC Cardiovasc Interv 2023;16(2):140–51.

37. Godino C, Munafò A, Scotti A, et al. MitraClip in secondary mitral regurgitation as a bridge to heart transplantation: 1-year outcomes from the International MitraBridge Registry. J Heart Lung Transplant 2020;39(12):1353–62.

38. Lim DS, Kar S, Spargias K, et al. Transcatheter Valve Repair for Patients With Mitral Regurgitation: 30-Day Results of the CLASP Study. JACC Cardiovasc Interv 2019;12(14):1369–78.

39. Webb JG, Hensey M, Szerlip M, et al. 1-Year Outcomes for Transcatheter Repair in Patients With Mitral Regurgitation From the CLASP Study. JACC Cardiovasc Interv 2020;13(20):2344–57.

40. Szerlip M, Spargias Konstantinos S, Makkar R, et al. 2-Year Outcomes for Transcatheter Repair in Patients With Mitral Regurgitation From the CLASP Study. JACC Cardiovasc Interv 2021;14(14): 1538–48.

41. Lim DS, Smith RL, Gillam LD, et al. Randomized Comparison of Transcatheter Edge-to-Edge Repair for Degenerative Mitral Regurgitation in Prohibitive Surgical Risk Patients. JACC Cardiovasc Interv 2022;15(24):2523–36.

42. Schneider L, Markovic S, Mueller K, et al. Mitral Valve Transcatheter Edge-to-Edge Repair Using MitraClip or PASCAL. JACC Cardiovasc Interv 2022; 15(24):2554–67.

43. Mauri V, Sugiura A, Spieker M, et al. Early Outcomes of 2 Mitral Valve Transcatheter Leaflet Approximation Devices: A Propensity Score-Matched Multicenter Comparison. JACC Cardiovasc Interv 2022;15(24): 2541–51.

44. Gerçek M, Roder F, Rudolph TK, et al. PASCAL mitral valve repair system versus MitraClip: comparison of transcatheter edge-to-edge strategies in complex primary mitral regurgitation. Clin Res Cardiol 2021;110(12):1890–9.

45. Sorajja P, Moat N, Badhwar V, et al. Initial Feasibility Study of a New Transcatheter Mitral Prosthesis: The First 100 Patients. J Am Coll Cardiol 2019;73(11): 1250–60.

46. Muller DWM, Farivar RS, Jansz P, et al. Transcatheter Mitral Valve Replacement for Patients With Symptomatic Mitral Regurgitation: A Global Feasibility Trial. J Am Coll Cardiol 2017;69(4):381–91.

47. Muller DWM, Sorajja P, Duncan A, et al. 2-Year Outcomes of Transcatheter Mitral Valve Replacement in Patients With Severe Symptomatic Mitral Regurgitation. J Am Coll Cardiol 2021;78(19):1847–59.

48. Wild MG, Kreidel F, Hell MM, et al. Transapical mitral valve implantation for treatment of symptomatic mitral valve disease: a real-world multicentre experience. Eur J Heart Fail 2022;24(5):899–907.

49. Ben Ali W, Ludwig S, Duncan A, et al. Characteristics and outcomes of patients screened for transcatheter mitral valve implantation: 1-year results from the CHOICE-MI registry. Eur J Heart Fail 2022;24(5):887–98.

50. Whisenant B, Kapadia SR, Eleid MF, et al. One-Year Outcomes of Mitral Valve-in-Valve Using the SAPIEN 3 Transcatheter Heart Valve. JAMA cardiology 2020; 5(11):1245–52.

51. Simonato M, Whisenant B, Ribeiro HB, et al. Transcatheter Mitral Valve Replacement After Surgical Repair or Replacement: Comprehensive Midterm Evaluation of Valve-in-Valve and Valve-in-Ring Implantation From the VIVID Registry. Circulation 2021;143(2):104–16.

Assessment of Right Ventricle Function and Tricuspid Regurgitation in Heart Failure: Current Advances in Diagnosis and Imaging

Vinesh Appadurai, MBBS[a,b], Taimur Safdur, MD[a], Akhil Narang, MD[a,*]

KEYWORDS

- Right ventricle • Tricuspid regurgitation • Heart failure • Cardiovascular imaging

KEY POINTS

- The right ventricle (RV) is an anatomically complex structure that often requires multimodality imaging for complete assessment.
- Tricuspid regurgitation quantitation can be performed across various imaging modalities.
- Advanced tissue tracking techniques can add value to quantifying RV function.
- Three-dimensional imaging is valuable, reproducible, and important for quantifying RV volumes and function.
- Promising advances in artificial intelligence can aide in imaging the RV and quantifying tricuspid regurgitation.

 Video content accompanies this article at http://www.heartfailure.theclinics.com.

INTRODUCTION

Heart failure is a complex clinical syndrome that carries significant morbidity and mortality.[1] The lifetime risk for heart failure remains high, with estimates ranging from 20% to 45% of the population after the age of 45 years, thus accounting for millions of heart failure presentations.[2] There are an array of pathophysiologic mechanisms that are involved in the genesis and evolution of heart failure.[3] The predominant cardiac chamber affected in heart failure syndromes is the left ventricle; however, approximately 50% of heart failure with reduced ejection fraction and over a third of heart failure with preserved ejection fraction presentations have concomitant right ventricle dysfunction (RVD).[4,5] Furthermore, right ventricle (RV) involvement in genetic, infiltrative, ischemic, and valvular myopathies are also prevalent.[6–11] Importantly, the presence of RVD carries a significantly poorer prognosis within these respective populations.[4,5,8–11]

The principal mechanism for RVD can be secondary to either significant volume loading, pressure overload, or intrinsic myocyte dysfunction and in some cases a combination of these.[12] Significant volume loading leading to RVD may occur

[a] Bluhm Cardiovascular Institute, Northwestern University, 676 North St Clair Street Suite 19-100 Galter Pavilion, Chicago, IL 60611, USA; [b] School of Medicine, The University of Queensland, St Lucia, QLD, 4067 Australia
* Corresponding author.
E-mail address: akhil.narang@nm.org

Heart Failure Clin 19 (2023) 317–328
https://doi.org/10.1016/j.hfc.2023.02.002
1551-7136/23/© 2023 Elsevier Inc. All rights reserved.

due to significant tricuspid regurgitation (TR) with compensatory RV dilatation occurring to ensure adequate preload demands are met.[13] Less commonly, significant volume loading may be due to preexisting large left-to-right-sided shunts. The most common cause of RV pressure overload results from acquired left-sided heart failure and secondly due to significant increases in pulmonary pressures from either primary lung disease or pulmonary thromboembolic phenomena.[12]

The geometric, hemodynamic, and functional mechanics of the right ventricle are important factors to take into consideration when determining the appropriate imaging modality for the initial assessment and subsequent monitoring of RVD.[14] In addition, the tricuspid valve (TV) structure and function is intimately involved in the hemodynamic and functional mechanics of the RV, and adequate consideration to the assessment of this valve is necessary.[15] This review focuses on the current landscape of imaging modalities and their value in the assessment of RVD and TR (**Table 1**) (**Fig. 1**).

ANATOMY OF THE RIGHT VENTRICLE AND TRICUSPID VALVE

Understanding the anatomy of the RV and TV is integral to appreciating the advantages and

disadvantages of the various noninvasive imaging modalities. The RV is the most anterior of the cardiac chambers and its shape can be described as a triangular hemisphere with a conal outflow tract in contrast to the prolated ellipsoid shape of the left ventricle.[12] The RV is heavily trabeculated and the contractile mechanics is more akin to a "bellows" motion in comparison to the multidimensional torsional, circumferential, shortening, and oblique contraction associated with the left ventricle.[16] Importantly, the RV may be delineated into three components: first, the RV inlet, which consists of the TV, chordae tendineae, and papillary muscles; second, the trabeculated apex; and finally the conus region that comprises the smooth outflow tract.[17] The RV walls are significantly thinner than the LV, measuring on average 2 to 5 mm in thickness.[16] The subendocardial fibers have a longitudinal configuration from the RV base to apex, whereas the subepicardial fibers have a circumferential arrangement that turn obliquely as they extend toward the apex with continuation on to the LV.[17] In addition, the RV septum plays an important contribution in the longitudinal shortening of the RV that occurs in systole and its continuation with the LV septum needs consideration when there is concomitant LV pathology.[12] The RV coronary artery territory is a low pressure and relatively compliant system

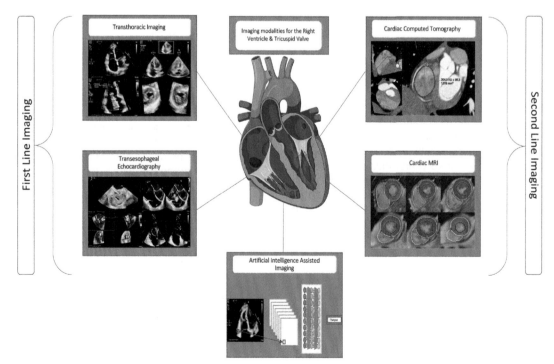

Fig. 1. Overview of important imaging modalities for assessing the right ventricle and quantifying tricuspid regurgitation. (Created with Biorender.com.)

Table 1
Multimodality comparison

	Echocardiography	CMR	CT
Advantages	• No radiation • High temporal and spatial resolution • Allows for functional and hemodynamic assessment • Readily available and portable	• No radiation • Gold standard for assessing ventricular size and function • Can assess for infiltrative disease in addition to ventricular and valvular dysfunction (tissue characterization)	• Gold standard for anatomical evaluation—high spatial resolution, adjacent structural evaluation, coronary anatomy
Disadvantages	• Body habitus can affect quality of images • Acoustic shadowing from prosthetic structures • Tradeoff between spatial and temporal resolution	• May not be as readily available • Patient claustrophobia • Relative cost • Artifact from prosthetic structures/intracardiac leads	• Radiation exposure • Artifact from calcified or prosthetic structures/intracardiac leads • Use of iodinated contrast

Abbreviations: CMR, cardiovascular MRI; CT, computed tomography.

that is predominantly supplied by the right coronary artery with the apical portion of the ventricle potentially being supplied from either or a combination of the right and left anterior descending coronary arteries.[18]

The TV anatomy is intimately affected by any alterations in RV anatomy. This is due to the four components of the TV that include the fibrous annulus attaching the TV to the right atrium and ventricle, the three leaflets (can be up to five), the papillary muscles, and the corresponding chordal attachments.[13,19] RVD alters the geometry and compliance of the fibrous annulus, papillary muscles, and chordal attachments and can therefore result in TV incompetence. Noninvasive imaging modalities thus have the challenge of needing to acquire the RV in planes that will be able accurately quantify ventricular volumes, myocardial wall thickness, ventricular functional changes, and consequent TV function. To date, there is no single imaging modality that can meet the complete demands of real-time imaging, ease of accessibility, comprehensive anatomical, hemodynamic, and perfusion assessment but instead a combination of modalities may be required for complete assessment.

Imaging the Right Heart

Echocardiography and the right ventricle

Echocardiography is often the first-line choice in assessing the RV due to its accessibility, affordability, reproducibility, and safety profile. Transthoracic echocardiography (TTE) can provide evaluation of RV structure, size, systolic function, and hemodynamic status. In addition, TTE can quantitate TV structure, function, and degree of regurgitation. There are well-established echocardiographic recommendations for the standardized assessment of the RV and TV.[20,21]

Two-dimensional (2D) echocardiography has supplanted M-mode based imaging and has furthered our understanding of the complex geometric nature of the RV. Guideline recommendations advocate the use of standardized linear dimensions for measuring the RV base, mid–ventricle, and base to apex length.[20] Limitations to this involve the significant variability in linear measurements with minor probe manipulation and the lack of spatial resolution when compared with cardiac MRI.[22] Genovese and colleagues[22] demonstrated significant interoperator variability in assessing RV dimensions in the traditional apical four-chamber view but improved quantification in the RV-focused view with the least variability. Additional windows such as the parasternal long-axis and parasternal short-axis views can add confirmatory information to the apical views obtained.[20] However, these views also do not incorporate the complex volumetric contribution of the right ventricular outflow (RVOT), which can contribute up to 20% of the RV volume.[23] More recently, the World Alliance Societies of Echocardiography have published international data for standardized values of RV dimensions, and these have more comprehensive multiracial data compared with the original dimensions included in guidelines that focused primarily on Caucasian populations.[24,25] Of note, the upper limit of normal ranges seems to be lower for RV dimensions and the lower limit of normal ranges for systolic function parameters seem to be higher than guideline recommendations (**Table 2**).[20,24,25] However, it is yet to be determined, how these new data will affect forthcoming guidelines, reporting recommendations, and predicting heart failure outcomes. Even taking these changes into consideration, 2D linear measurements fail to capture the unique functional mechanics of the RV, which is important for patients at risk of and with heart failure.[26] To address these inherent short-comings, a novel three-dimensional (3D) echocardiography and speckle-tracking echocardiography have added significant value to volumetric assessments of the RV and functional quantitation, respectively.[27,28]

Three-dimensional echocardiography functions through the acquisition of full-volume pyramidal data sets that incorporate the complete dimensions of the RV.[29] The normative values of RV volumes with 3D data sets are available but underestimate and demonstrate modest correlations when compared with cardiac MRI volumes.[30,31] However, 3D right ventricle ejection fraction (RVEF) has very good correlations with cardiac MRI.[32,33] The 3D RVEF and dimensions have demonstrable value over traditional linear dimensions as a predictor of clinical outcomes in RV dysfunction and heart failure.[27,34–37] Limitations to 3D RV assessments are the dependence on the quality of 2D images and available acoustic windows.[38] In addition, in RV dilatation, there can be difficulty in full acquisition of the RV free wall or anterior walls due to limitations in pyramidal data set acquisitions, and therefore, 3D echocardiography may not be possible in all patients.[38]

Although acoustic windows may limit visualization of the RV endocardial border, options for managing these cases may include the utility of ultrasound-enhancing agents (UEAs) which have been used with great success to optimize 2D imaging of the RV when there is significant shadowing.[39]

UEAs are composed of compressible microbubbles containing high-molecular weight gases that provide better blood pool to endocardial border differentiation and provide greater correlation with cardiac MRI-derived volumes.[39] Furthermore, the combination of UEAs and 3D echocardiography has been previously investigated with significant improvement in endocardial borders and an accuracy of 3D volumes.[40]

The assessment of RV function is particularly relevant to heart failure diagnosis and monitoring. There are several parameters that can be used for RV systolic function quantitation in addition to 3D RVEF. Traditional parameters that have demonstrated prognostic value and are recommended in standard transthoracic acquisition are the RV S' (S prime), tricuspid annular plane systolic excursion (TAPSE), and fractional area change (FAC).[41] More comprehensive parameters include 2D RV free wall strain (2D-RV FWS), 2D RV global strain (2D-RV GLS), 3D RV strain (3D RVS), and RV myocardial performance index.[41] Strain measurements are dimensionless and performed with speckle-tracking echocardiography, quantifying deformation of myocardial tissue through tracking of reflected echo speckles.[42] Impairments in RV S', TAPSE, and FAC are all established predictors of RV failure and are associated with prognostic outcomes in a variety of respiratory pathologies, RV myopathies, and left-sided heart disease.[43,44] However, 2D RV FWS, RV GLS, and 3D RVS provide incrementally superior value over tissue Doppler parameters for prognosis in heart failure patients.[42,45] In addition, they are more sensitive markers of RVD in pulmonary hypertension secondary to any cause and RV-specific myopathies.[45,46]

When comparing RV 2D strain with 3D strain, it should be noted that 2D RV FWS is easily taught, performed, reproducible and can be retrospectively applied in standardized RV views compared with 3D RVS, which requires the specific acquisition of 3D RV data sets limiting its application in

Table 2				
Right ventricle size and functional normal values[21,91–93]				
	Echocardiogram		CMR	
Variable	Men	Women	Men	Women
RV EDV (mL/m²)	35–87	32–74	58–109	51–97
RV ESV (mL/m²)	10–44	8–36	12–46	9–42
RVEF (%)	>45 (3D)		51–80	
RVFW strain (%)	< −20		—	

Abbreviations: EDV, end diastolic volume; ESV, end systolic volume; RV, right ventricle; RVEF, right ventricle ejection fraction; RVFW, right ventricle free wall.

a significant proportion of cases.[29,47] Furthermore, there is significantly more data available verifying the functional and prognostic value of 2D FWS when compared with that available for 3D RVS in heart failure patients.[42]

RV to pulmonary artery (RV-PA) coupling is an important relationship between RV contractility and RV afterload.[48] RV contractility should match afterload (in the form of PA pressures), and therefore, they are coupled from a physiologic perspective.[48] If RV afterload increases, RV contractility should also in turn escalate to compensate for the elevations in pressures to thus maintain satisfactory global RV function. When RV contractility starts to decline due to significant increases in RV afterload or prolonged exposure to high afterload, this results in RV-PA uncoupling and is a poor prognostic marker for patients in which pulmonary hypertension is present.[48] Noninvasive measures of RV-PA coupling can be quantified through echocardiography and the measure of TAPSE or RV FWS divided by PA systolic pressures can yield valuable and prognostic information on RV-PA coupling within heart failure populations.[49–52]

Transesophageal echocardiography (TEE) can provide some additional information to RV volume and function acquisition due to its clearer imaging windows of the RV. Unlike TTE, TEE has unhindered acoustic windows of the complete RV free wall and there is the option for 3D volumetric acquisitions of the complete RV. 2D RVFWS can also be acquired and add significant information for global RV function, particularly when TEE Doppler parameters are not easily obtainable due to poor probe alignment. Limitations to TEE acquisitions of RV function are the volumetric and hemodynamic changes that occur with sedation required to perform TEEs.[53] Consequentially, RV function may be underestimated due to reductions in function from these conditions required for TEE.[53]

The value of echocardiography in tricuspid regurgitation

Echocardiography is the primary imaging modality for the assessment of TR severity.[21] The higher temporal resolution and ability to assess hemodynamics through Doppler principles allow reliable quantitation, localization, and mechanism of TR.[21] Color Doppler detection of regurgitant jets combined with pulsed and continuous wave Doppler interrogation allows volumetric quantitation of jet flow through harnessing fundamental principles of conservation of mass, flow, and momentum (see **Fig. 3**).[54] Reference values for echocardiographic-based TR severity can be found in **Table 3**. Isolated and combined severe

TR is associated with poor outcomes in a variety of populations, including postsurgical patients. TR in heart failure is predominantly secondary to a functional etiology which can be due to RV dilatation, RV or pulmonary hypertension, annular dilatation, or regional or global RV failure.[13] TTE can identify these causes from 2D imaging and assessment of pulmonary pressures.[13] Recent work by Akintoye and colleagues,[55] investigating echocardiographic predictors in asymptomatic severe TR patients, has identified TTE-defined regurgitant volumes greater than 45 mL and RV FWS less than 19% as predictive cutoffs for increased all-cause mortality and may provide important guidance for intervention in this challenging cohort. More recently, significant interest has been directed toward the morphological determination of tricuspid leaflet anatomy and localization of regurgitation as the field of transcatheter interventional options for this valve is expanding.[19,54] The 3D echocardiography in TTE imaging can also aide in determining and localizing TR; however, the spatial resolution is significantly reduced when compared with TEE 3D imaging due to the TV appearing in the far field.[38] The TEE imaging of the TV is an important adjunct to TTE imaging and excels in the quantitation, localization, and mechanism of TR. This is due to the improved spatial resolution as the TV is closer to the probe and rib shadowing and limited acoustic windows are not factors. TEE imaging is also required for any preplanning of structural interventions on the TV as imaging guidance is integral for currently available transcatheter valve interventions. The limitations of TEE imaging include the negative effects of procedural sedation on preload which may result in underestimation of TR severity.[53,56] Importantly, echocardiographic-derived indices of TR severity, including proximal isovelocity surface area (PISA), effective regurgitant orifice area (EROA), jet size to chamber ratios, and regurgitant volume quantitation are all associated with clinical and remodeling outcomes.[57,58]

Cardiac MRI in imaging the right ventricle and tricuspid regurgitation

Cardiac MRI is the gold-standard imaging modality for determining RV volumes, RV geometry, and tissue characterization.[59] The standardized protocol for scanning the RV in cardiac MRI involves cine imaging from multiple planes including inflow, outflow, and short axis cine stack. Additional T1- and T2-weighted sequences and late gadolinium enhancement sequences allow for tissue characterization.[60] Short-axis stacks of the RV also allow for evaluation of RV radial and circumferential

Table 3
Tricuspid regurgitation severity grading

Imaging Modality		TR Severity Grading				
		Mild	Moderate	Severe	Massive	Torrential
Echocardiography[54]	VCW (cm²)	<0.3	0.3–0.69	≥0.7	—	—
	PISA (cm³)	≤0.5	0.6–0.9	>0.9	—	—
	EROA (cm²)	<0.20	0.20–0.395	≥0.40	—	—
	Rvol (2D PISA) (mL)	<30	30–44	≥45	—	—
	3D VC (mm²)	—	—	75–94	95–114	≥115
CMR[91]	RF (%)	≤15	16–25	26–48	—	—

Abbreviations: CWD, continuous wave Doppler; EROA, effective regurgitant orifice area; PISA, proximal isovelocity surface area; RF, regurgitant fraction; VC, vena contracta; VCW, vena contracta width.

contraction which is not possible with TTE.[60] Owing to the thin-walled nature of the RV, there are limitations on cardiac MRI to formally quantitate fibrosis; however, semi-quantitative and qualitative analysis with LGE imaging can still be carried out to identify an infiltrative, inflammatory, or ischemic pattern distribution.[61] Fat suppression imaging can additionally be used for determining fatty infiltration and metaplasia for patients with suspected arrhythmogenic RV cardiomyopathy (ARVC).[60] Furthermore, advances in tissue tracking techniques allows for RV strain quantitation through feature tracking or tagging analysis.[62] These differ from echocardiographic-derived speckle-tracking imaging and have lower temporal resolution but there is a growing body of evidence for the diagnostic and prognostic value of feature tracking strain in RV myopathic processes.[63,64] The superior spatial resolution of cardiac MRI over echocardiography allows a more comprehensive 3D analysis with novel MRI-derived 3D volumetric rendering producing complex, reliable, and reproducible evaluations of the RV in patients with progressive RV failure, atypical morphologies, and patients with congenital heart disease.[65,66] Normative values for cardiac MRI-derived 3D volumes and ejection fractions are available for reference (see **Table 2**).[67]

Cardiac MRI can also provide incremental utility for TR severity quantitation through its superior measures of RV volumes over echocardiography.[68] However, some discrepancies may occur between cardiac MRI and echocardiographic-derived TR severities, with usually a 1 grade differential of severity occurring between them.[69] Volumetric determinations of severity can be used in conjunction with echocardiography to confirm severe TR as well as localize and reconstruct TV geometry to aide in determining the etiology of TR.[70] In heart failure with severely dilated RVs, this can prove useful, as a complete assessment of the RV is possible without the limitations of acoustic windows and

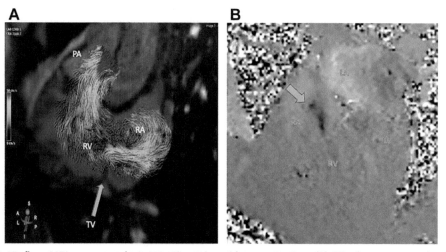

Fig. 2. (*A*) 4D flow MRI sequence demonstrating tricuspid regurgitation, (*B*) 2D phase contrast in plane MRI sequence of four-chamber view demonstrating tricuspid regurgitation (*arrow*). LV, left ventricle; PA, pulmonary artery; RA, right atrium; RV, right ventricle; TV, tricuspid valve.

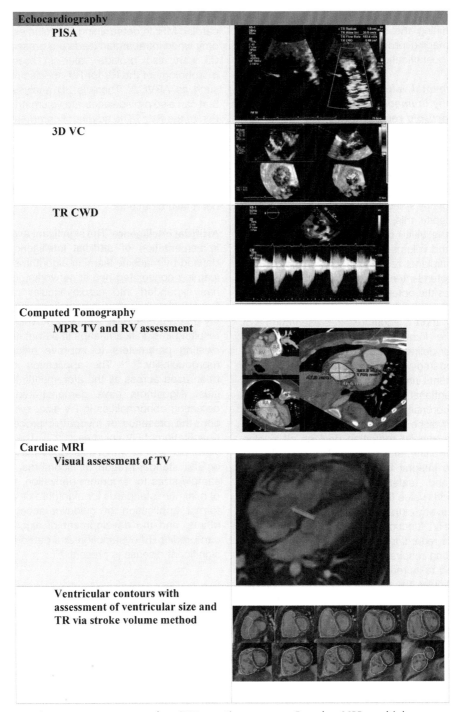

Fig. 3. TR severity measurement examples. CWD, continuous wave Doppler; MPR, multiplanar reconstruction; PISA, proximal isovelocity surface area; RA, right atrium; RV, right ventricle; TR, tricuspid regurgitation; TV, tricuspid valve; VC, vena contracta. Tricuspid valve (*arrow*).

shadowing.[54] There is evidence to also support the prognostic role of cardiac MRI in conjunction with echocardiographic-derived parameters in patients with isolated TR.[71] Recent advances in volumetric 4D flow quantification have added a new paradigm

to the assessment of TR by providing highly reproducible measures compared with multiplanar MRI but is still an area requiring more validation before clinical utility (**Fig. 2**, Videos 1 and 2).[72] Furthermore, cardiac MRI-derived stroke volume assessment is a recognized confirmatory method for determining the severity of TR with phase contrast imaging providing significant additional value as a quantification methodology.[21]

The incremental value of cardiac computed tomography in imaging the right ventricle and place in tricuspid regurgitation

Cardiac computed tomography (CT) is an ever evolving and readily accessible imaging modality for the anatomical assessment of cardiac structure.[73] The historic utility of cardiac CT is in the analysis of coronary artery distribution and the presence of any stenosis or anatomical abnormalities.[73] Despite this, there have been developments in the utility of cardiac CT in quantifying RV sizes and volumes, and provision of excellent spatial multiplanar reconstructions of the RV and TV for structural interventional preplanning.[74] Cardiac CT has the potential for reconstruction along multiple planes with greater spatial resolution providing more accurate representation of commissure locations, leaflet tenting heights, and greater delineation of the sub-valvular apparatus compared with TEE (**Fig. 3**).[74] RV annular measurements are also a crucial component of pre-interventional planning due to the course of the right coronary artery and its proximity with the annular plane. Emerging transcatheter TV implants and annular reduction devices all involve the annular plane, and precise planning with cardiac CT is integral to device suitability, performance, and safety.[75,76] Furthermore, this modality adds value through its ability to delineate pathology in any extra-cardiac organs that may be affecting RV function.[77] Cardiac CT provides information regarding the presence and severity of preexisting respiratory pathology that may be contributing to increased pressure loading on the RV. In particular, the presence of acute or chronic thromboembolic arterial/veno-occlusive disease, interstitial lung disease, or other significant respiratory causes of pulmonary hypertension. Cardiac CT can also identify anomalous venous or arterial malformations that may result in significant RV volume-loading conditions and the presence of anatomical shunts.[78]

Cardiac CT has demonstrable efficacy in measuring RV volumes.[79] Maffei and colleagues[80] demonstrated good correlation of 79 patients who underwent cardiac CT-derived RV volumes and RV EF when compared with cardiac MRI as the gold standard. Furthermore, a meta-analysis by Kim and colleagues[77] reviewing 20 studies with 766 patients found pooled correlation coefficients of $r = 0.87–0.93$ for all volumetric-based RV parameters when compared with cardiac MRI.

Particularly, useful is the utility of cardiac CT over cardiac MRI in determining RV volumes and anatomy when intracardiac leads are present. Cardiac CT can also provide value in assessing the morphology of the RV for RV-specific myopathies such as ARVC.[81] There is 3D analysis software that can also provide accurate volumetric quantitation of the RV.[77] The advent of commercially available cardiac CT strain analysis software has also provided another way to better quantify LV longitudinal and circumferential systolic function.[82] However, its utility in the RV has yet to be described but may provide promise for prognostication in heart failure patients.

Artificial intelligence The significant evolution and implementation of artificial intelligence (AI), as defined by machine learning algorithms and deep learning convoluted neural networks, in medicine has expanded into cardiovascular medicine.[83] Specifically, the utility of neural networks to identify and automatically segment moving images is resulting in significant leaps in automation of pre-existing parameters to improve efficiency and reproducibility.[84,85] The application of AI has been used across all the aforementioned modalities. Algorithms have demonstrated value in detecting abnormalities in RV size, systolic function, the presence of myopathic processes, and quantitation of RV volumes.[30,86–91] The future developments of AI within this space will likely focus on the standardization of algorithms, improving sample sizes for algorithm derivation, the setting of minimum standards for algorithm development, formal application of guideline-accepted algorithms, and the development of algorithms that can predict RV dysfunction and pathology before significant disease is present.[83]

SUMMARY

RV function is an important part of heart failure presentations. TR usually complicates these presentations and quantifying these two entities is integral in risk-stratifying heart failure patients. RV anatomy and function are complex and may require different modalities to provide comprehensive quantitation in particular cases. Echocardiography is the first-line imaging tool for RV assessment and TR quantitation, followed by cardiac MRI and/or cardiac CT when the need arises. Progress in 3D imaging in all three modalities has yielded improved quantitation of volumes and ejection fraction. Furthermore, advances in tissue-tracking strain and AI are promising for future applications in RV functional assessment and TR quantitation.

CLINICS CARE POINTS

- Echocardiography is the first-line imaging modality for the assessment of right ventricle (RV) structure and function, providing valuable diagnostic and prognostic information for clinical decision-making.
- Cardiac MRI and cardiac computed tomography (CT) play complementary roles in further defining the myopathic characteristics of the RV as well as formally quantifying RV volumes and ejection fraction.
- Tricuspid regurgitation is best initially quantified with transthoracic echocardiography and subsequently further defined by transesophageal echocardiography.
- Cardiac MRI and cardiac CT play important roles in determining regurgitant fractions and prestructural intervention planning, respectively.
- Artificial intelligence may play an important role in the future for confirming abnormal appearances, volumes, and function of the RV and alerting readers to the presence of tricuspid regurgitation that may benefit from intervention.

FUNDING

This research did not receive any specific grant from funding agencies in the public, commercial, or not-for-profit sectors.

ACKNOWLEDGEMENT

We acknowledge the Feis Foundation for providing funding to Dr Narang.

DISCLOSURES

None.

SUPPLEMENTARY DATA

Supplementary data related to this article can be found online at https://doi.org/10.1016/j.hfc.2023.02.002.

REFERENCES

1. Savarese G, Lund LH. Global public health burden of heart failure. Card Fail Rev 2017;3:7–11.
2. Tsao CW, Aday AW, Almarzooq ZI, et al. Heart disease and stroke statistics-2022 update: a report from the American Heart Association. Circulation 2022;145:e153–639.
3. Kemp CD, Conte JV. The pathophysiology of heart failure. Cardiovasc Pathol 2012;21:365–71.
4. Iglesias-Garriz I, Olalla-Gomez C, Garrote C, et al. Contribution of right ventricular dysfunction to heart failure mortality: a meta-analysis. Rev Cardiovasc Med 2012;13:e62–9.
5. Mohammed SF, Hussain I, AbouEzzeddine OF, et al. Right ventricular function in heart failure with preserved ejection fraction: a community-based study. Circulation 2014;130:2310–20.
6. Seo J, Hong YJ, Kim YJ, et al. Prevalence, functional characteristics, and clinical significance of right ventricular involvement in patients with hypertrophic cardiomyopathy. Sci Rep 2020;10:21908.
7. Bodez D, Ternacle J, Guellich A, et al. Prognostic value of right ventricular systolic function in cardiac amyloidosis. Amyloid 2016;23:158–67.
8. Gulati A, Ismail TF, Jabbour A, et al. The prevalence and prognostic significance of right ventricular systolic dysfunction in nonischemic dilated cardiomyopathy. Circulation 2013;128:1623–33.
9. Merlo M, Gobbo M, Stolfo D, et al. The prognostic impact of the evolution of RV function in idiopathic DCM. JACC Cardiovasc Imaging 2016;9:1034–42.
10. Dietz MF, Prihadi EA, van der Bijl P, et al. Prognostic implications of right ventricular remodeling and function in patients with significant secondary tricuspid regurgitation. Circulation 2019;140:836–45.
11. Dini FL, Conti U, Fontanive P, et al. Right ventricular dysfunction is a major predictor of outcome in patients with moderate to severe mitral regurgitation and left ventricular dysfunction. Am Heart J 2007;154:172–9.
12. Sanz J, Sanchez-Quintana D, Bossone E, et al. Anatomy, function, and dysfunction of the right ventricle: JACC state-of-the-art review. J Am Coll Cardiol 2019;73:1463–82.
13. Hahn RT. State-of-the-art review of echocardiographic imaging in the evaluation and treatment of functional tricuspid regurgitation. Circ Cardiovasc Imaging 2016;9:e005332.
14. Jones N, Burns AT, Prior DL. Echocardiographic assessment of the right ventricle-state of the art. Heart Lung Circ 2019;28:1339–50.
15. Rana BS, Robinson S, Francis R, et al. Tricuspid regurgitation and the right ventricle in risk stratification and timing of intervention. Echo Res Pract 2019;6:R25–39.
16. Ho SY, Nihoyannopoulos P. Anatomy, echocardiography, and normal right ventricular dimensions. Heart 2006;92(Suppl 1):i2–13.
17. Haddad F, Hunt SA, Rosenthal DN, et al. Right ventricular function in cardiovascular disease, part I: anatomy, physiology, aging, and functional assessment of the right ventricle. Circulation 2008;117:1436–48.

18. Crystal GJ, Pagel PS. Right ventricular perfusion: physiology and clinical implications. Anesthesiology 2018;128:202–18.

19. Hahn RT, Weckbach LT, Noack T, et al. Proposal for a standard echocardiographic tricuspid valve nomenclature. JACC Cardiovasc Imaging 2021;14:1299–305.

20. Rudski LG, Lai WW, Afilalo J, et al. Guidelines for the echocardiographic assessment of the right heart in adults: a report from the American Society of Echocardiography endorsed by the European Association of Echocardiography, a registered branch of the European Society of Cardiology, and the Canadian Society of Echocardiography. J Am Soc Echocardiogr 2010;23:685–713 [quiz: 786-8].

21. Zoghbi WA, Adams D, Bonow RO, et al. Recommendations for noninvasive evaluation of native valvular regurgitation: a report from the American society of echocardiography developed in collaboration with the society for cardiovascular magnetic resonance. J Am Soc Echocardiogr 2017;30:303–71.

22. Genovese D, Mor-Avi V, Palermo C, et al. Comparison between four-chamber and right ventricular-focused views for the quantitative evaluation of right ventricular size and function. J Am Soc Echocardiogr 2019;32:484–94.

23. Geva T, Powell AJ, Crawford EC, et al. Evaluation of regional differences in right ventricular systolic function by acoustic quantification echocardiography and cine magnetic resonance imaging. Circulation 1998;98:339–45.

24. Addetia K, Miyoshi T, Citro R, et al. Two-dimensional echocardiographic right ventricular size and systolic function measurements stratified by sex, age, and ethnicity: results of the world alliance of societies of echocardiography study. J Am Soc Echocardiogr 2021;34:1148–1157 e1.

25. Soulat-Dufour L, Addetia K, Miyoshi T, et al. Normal values of right atrial size and function according to age, sex, and ethnicity: results of the world alliance societies of echocardiography study. J Am Soc Echocardiogr 2021;34:286–300.

26. Gripari P, Muratori M, Fusini L, et al. Right ventricular dimensions and function: why do we need a more accurate and quantitative imaging? J Cardiovasc Echogr 2015;25:19–25.

27. Nagata Y, Wu VC, Kado Y, et al. Prognostic value of right ventricular ejection fraction assessed by transthoracic 3D echocardiography. Circ Cardiovasc Imaging 2017;10:e005384.

28. Carluccio E, Biagioli P, Alunni G, et al. Prognostic value of right ventricular dysfunction in heart failure with reduced ejection fraction: superiority of longitudinal strain over tricuspid annular plane systolic excursion. Circ Cardiovasc Imaging 2018;11:e006894.

29. Shiota T. 3D echocardiography: evaluation of the right ventricle. Curr Opin Cardiol 2009;24:410–4.

30. Zhu Y, Bao Y, Zheng K, et al. Quantitative assessment of right ventricular size and function with multiple parameters from artificial intelligence-based three-dimensional echocardiography: a comparative study with cardiac magnetic resonance. Echocardiography 2022;39:223–32.

31. Greiner S, Andre F, Heimisch M, et al. A closer look at right ventricular 3D volume quantification by transthoracic echocardiography and cardiac MRI. Clin Radiol 2019;74:490 e7–490 e14.

32. Wang S, Wang S, Zhu Q, et al. Reference values of right ventricular volumes and ejection fraction by three-dimensional echocardiography in adults: a systematic review and meta-analysis. Front Cardiovasc Med 2021;8:709863.

33. Otani K, Nabeshima Y, Kitano T, et al. Accuracy of fully automated right ventricular quantification software with 3D echocardiography: direct comparison with cardiac magnetic resonance and semi-automated quantification software. Eur Heart J Cardiovasc Imaging 2020;21:787–95.

34. Meng Y, Zhu S, Xie Y, et al. Prognostic value of right ventricular 3D speckle-tracking strain and ejection fraction in patients with HFpEF. Front Cardiovasc Med 2021;8:694365.

35. Zhang Y, Sun W, Wu C, et al. Prognostic value of right ventricular ejection fraction assessed by 3D echocardiography in COVID-19 patients. Front Cardiovasc Med 2021;8:641088.

36. Magunia H, Dietrich C, Langer HF, et al. 3D echocardiography derived right ventricular function is associated with right ventricular failure and mid-term survival after left ventricular assist device implantation. Int J Cardiol 2018;272:348–55.

37. Muraru D, Badano LP, Nagata Y, et al. Development and prognostic validation of partition values to grade right ventricular dysfunction severity using 3D echocardiography. Eur Heart J Cardiovasc Imaging 2020;21:10–21.

38. Lang RM, Addetia K, Narang A, et al. 3-dimensional echocardiography: latest developments and future directions. JACC Cardiovasc Imaging 2018;11:1854–78.

39. Porter TR, Mulvagh SL, Abdelmoneim SS, et al. Clinical applications of ultrasonic enhancing agents in echocardiography: 2018 american society of echocardiography guidelines update. J Am Soc Echocardiogr 2018;31:241–74.

40. Medvedofsky D, Mor-Avi V, Kruse E, et al. Quantification of right ventricular size and function from contrast-enhanced three-dimensional echocardiographic images. J Am Soc Echocardiogr 2017;30:1193–202.

41. Mitchell C, Rahko PS, Blauwet LA, et al. Guidelines for performing a comprehensive transthoracic echocardiographic examination in adults: recommendations from the american society of echocardiography. J Am Soc Echocardiogr 2019;32:1–64.

42. Muraru D, Haugaa K, Donal E, et al. Right ventricular longitudinal strain in the clinical routine: a state-of-the-art review. Eur Heart J Cardiovasc Imaging 2022;23:898–912.

43. Bistola V, Parissis JT, Paraskevaidis I, et al. Prognostic value of tissue Doppler right ventricular systolic and diastolic function indexes combined with plasma B-type natriuretic Peptide in patients with advanced heart failure secondary to ischemic or idiopathic dilated cardiomyopathy. Am J Cardiol 2010;105:249–54.

44. Anavekar NS, Skali H, Bourgoun M, et al. Usefulness of right ventricular fractional area change to predict death, heart failure, and stroke following myocardial infarction (from the VALIANT ECHO Study). Am J Cardiol 2008;101:607–12.

45. Hulshof HG, Eijsvogels TMH, Kleinnibbelink G, et al. Prognostic value of right ventricular longitudinal strain in patients with pulmonary hypertension: a systematic review and meta-analysis. Eur Heart J Cardiovasc Imaging 2019;20:475–84.

46. Fine NM, Chen L, Bastiansen PM, et al. Outcome prediction by quantitative right ventricular function assessment in 575 subjects evaluated for pulmonary hypertension. Circ Cardiovasc Imaging 2013;6:711–21.

47. Chamberlain R, Scalia GM, Wee Y, et al. The learning curve for competency in right ventricular longitudinal strain analysis. J Am Soc Echocardiogr 2020;33:512–4.

48. Sathananthan G, Grewal J. The complex relationship That Is RV-PA coupling and its relevance to managing congenital heart disease. Can J Cardiol 2019;35:816–8.

49. Jentzer JC, Anavekar NS, Reddy YNV, et al. Right ventricular pulmonary artery coupling and mortality in cardiac intensive care unit patients. J Am Heart Assoc 2021;10:e019015.

50. Tello K, Axmann J, Ghofrani HA, et al. Relevance of the TAPSE/PASP ratio in pulmonary arterial hypertension. Int J Cardiol 2018;266:229–35.

51. Unlu S, Bezy S, Cvijic M, et al. Right ventricular strain related to pulmonary artery pressure predicts clinical outcome in patients with pulmonary arterial hypertension. Eur Heart J Cardiovasc Imaging 2022;19:jeac136.

52. Brener MI, Grayburn P, Lindenfeld J, et al. Right ventricular-pulmonary arterial coupling in patients with HF Secondary MR: analysis from the COAPT trial. JACC Cardiovasc Interv 2021;14:2231–42.

53. Magunia H, Jordanow A, Keller M, et al. The effects of anesthesia induction and positive pressure ventilation on right-ventricular function: an echocardiography-based prospective observational study. BMC Anesthesiol 2019;19:199.

54. Hahn RT, Thomas JD, Khalique OK, et al. Imaging assessment of tricuspid regurgitation severity. JACC Cardiovasc Imaging 2019;12:469–90.

55. Akintoye E, Wang TKM, Nakhla M, et al. Quantitative echocardiographic assessment and optimal criteria for early intervention in asymptomatic tricuspid regurgitation. JACC Cardiovasc Imaging 2023;16(1):13–24.

56. Antunes MJ, Rodriguez-Palomares J, Prendergast B, et al. Management of tricuspid valve regurgitation: Position statement of the European society of cardiology working groups of cardiovascular surgery and valvular heart disease. Eur J Cardio Thorac Surg 2017;52:1022–30.

57. Bannehr M, Edlinger CR, Kahn U, et al. Natural course of tricuspid regurgitation and prognostic implications. Open Heart 2021;8:e001529.

58. Topilsky Y, Inojosa JM, Benfari G, et al. Clinical presentation and outcome of tricuspid regurgitation in patients with systolic dysfunction. Eur Heart J 2018;39:3584–92.

59. Benza R, Biederman R, Murali S, et al. Role of cardiac magnetic resonance imaging in the management of patients with pulmonary arterial hypertension. J Am Coll Cardiol 2008;52:1683–92.

60. Kramer CM, Barkhausen J, Bucciarelli-Ducci C, et al. Standardized cardiovascular magnetic resonance imaging (CMR) protocols: 2020 update. J Cardiovasc Magn Reson 2020;22:17.

61. Mewton N, Liu CY, Croisille P, et al. Assessment of myocardial fibrosis with cardiovascular magnetic resonance. J Am Coll Cardiol 2011;57:891–903.

62. Erley J, Tanacli R, Genovese D, et al. Myocardial strain analysis of the right ventricle: comparison of different cardiovascular magnetic resonance and echocardiographic techniques. J Cardiovasc Magn Reson 2020;22:51.

63. Romano S, Dell'atti D, Judd RM, et al. Prognostic Value of feature-tracking right ventricular longitudinal strain in severe functional tricuspid regurgitation: a multicenter study. JACC Cardiovasc Imaging 2021;14:1561–8.

64. Bourfiss M, Prakken NHJ, James CA, et al. Prognostic value of strain by feature-tracking cardiac magnetic resonance in arrhythmogenic right ventricular cardiomyopathy. Eur Heart J Cardiovasc Imaging 2022;24(1):98–107.

65. Goo HW. Comparison between three-dimensional navigator-gated whole-heart MRI and two-dimensional cine MRI in quantifying ventricular volumes. Korean J Radiol 2018;19:704–14.

66. Uribe S, Tangchaoren T, Parish V, et al. Volumetric cardiac quantification by using 3D dual-phase whole-heart MR imaging. Radiology 2008;248:606–14.

67. Maceira AM, Prasad SK, Khan M, et al. Normalized left ventricular systolic and diastolic function by steady state free precession cardiovascular magnetic resonance. J Cardiovasc Magn Reson 2006;8:417–26.

68. Medvedofsky D, Leon Jimenez J, Addetia K, et al. Multi-parametric quantification of tricuspid regurgitation using cardiovascular magnetic resonance: a

comparison to echocardiography. Eur J Radiol 2017;86:213–20.

69. Zhan Y, Senapati A, Vejpongsa P, et al. Comparison of echocardiographic assessment of tricuspid regurgitation against cardiovascular magnetic resonance. JACC Cardiovasc Imaging 2020;13:1461–71.

70. Saremi F, Hassani C, Millan-Nunez V, et al. Imaging evaluation of tricuspid valve: analysis of morphology and function with CT and MRI. AJR Am J Roentgenol 2015;204:W531–42.

71. Wang TKM, Akyuz K, Reyaldeen R, et al. Prognostic value of complementary echocardiography and magnetic resonance imaging quantitative evaluation for isolated tricuspid regurgitation. Circ Cardiovasc Imaging 2021;14:e012211.

72. Feneis JF, Kyubwa E, Atianzar K, et al. 4D flow MRI quantification of mitral and tricuspid regurgitation: Reproducibility and consistency relative to conventional MRI. J Magn Reson Imaging 2018;48:1147–58.

73. Abdelrahman KM, Chen MY, Dey AK, et al. Coronary computed tomography angiography from clinical uses to emerging technologies: JACC state-of-the-art review. J Am Coll Cardiol 2020;76:1226–43.

74. Pulerwitz TC, Khalique OK, Leb J, et al. Optimizing cardiac CT Protocols for comprehensive acquisition prior to percutaneous MV and TV repair/replacement. JACC Cardiovasc Imaging 2020;13:836–50.

75. Gray WA, Abramson SV, Lim S, et al. 1-year outcomes of cardioband tricuspid valve reconstruction system early feasibility study. JACC Cardiovasc Interv 2022;15:1921–32.

76. Webb JG, Chuang AM, Meier D, et al. Transcatheter tricuspid valve replacement with the EVOQUE system: 1-year outcomes of a multicenter, first-in-human experience. JACC Cardiovasc Interv 2022;15:481–91.

77. Kim JY, Suh YJ, Han K, et al. Cardiac CT for measurement of right ventricular volume and function in comparison with cardiac MRI: a meta-analysis. Korean J Radiol 2020;21:450–61.

78. Dillman JR, Hernandez RJ. Role of CT in the evaluation of congenital cardiovascular disease in children. AJR Am J Roentgenol 2009;192:1219–31.

79. Sugeng L, Mor-Avi V, Weinert L, et al. Multimodality comparison of quantitative volumetric analysis of the right ventricle. JACC Cardiovasc Imaging 2010;3:10–8.

80. Maffei E, Messalli G, Martini C, et al. Left and right ventricle assessment with Cardiac CT: validation study vs. Cardiac MR. Eur Radiol 2012;22:1041–9.

81. Tandri H, Calkins H. MR and CT imaging of arrhythmogenic cardiomyopathy. Card Electrophysiol Clin 2011;3:269–80.

82. Marwan M, Ammon F, Bittner D, et al. CT-derived left ventricular global strain in aortic valve stenosis patients: a comparative analysis pre and post transcatheter aortic valve implantation. J Cardiovasc Comput Tomogr 2018;12:240–4.

83. Dey D, Slomka PJ, Leeson P, et al. Artificial intelligence in cardiovascular imaging: JACC State-of-the-Art Review. J Am Coll Cardiol 2019;73:1317–35.

84. Kusunose K, Haga A, Abe T, et al. Utilization of artificial intelligence in echocardiography. Circ J 2019;83:1623–9.

85. Kusunose K, Haga A, Inoue M, et al. Clinically feasible and accurate view classification of echocardiographic images using deep learning. Biomolecules 2020;10:665.

86. Ahmad A, Ibrahim Z, Sakr G, et al. A comparison of artificial intelligence-based algorithms for the identification of patients with depressed right ventricular function from 2-dimentional echocardiography parameters and clinical features. Cardiovasc Diagn Ther 2020;10:859–68.

87. Wang S, Chauhan D, Patel H, et al. Assessment of right ventricular size and function from cardiovascular magnetic resonance images using artificial intelligence. J Cardiovasc Magn Reson 2022;24:27.

88. Alabed S, Alandejani F, Dwivedi K, et al. Validation of artificial intelligence cardiac MRI measurements: relationship to heart catheterization and mortality prediction. Radiology 2022;304:E56.

89. Genovese D, Rashedi N, Weinert L, et al. Machine learning-based three-dimensional echocardiographic quantification of right ventricular size and function: validation against cardiac magnetic resonance. J Am Soc Echocardiogr 2019;32:969–77.

90. Beecy AN, Bratt A, Yum B, et al. Development of novel machine learning model for right ventricular quantification on echocardiography-A multimodality validation study. Echocardiography 2020;37:688–97.

91. Medvedofsky D, Mor-Avi V, Amzulescu M, et al. Three-dimensional echocardiographic quantification of the left-heart chambers using an automated adaptive analytics algorithm: multicentre validation study. Eur Heart J Cardiovasc Imaging 2018;19:47–58.

92. Kawel-Boehm N, Hetzel SJ, Ambale-Venkatesh B, et al. Reference ranges ("normal values") for cardiovascular magnetic resonance (CMR) in adults and children: 2020 update. J Cardiovasc Magn Reson 2020;22:87.

93. Lang RM, Badano LP, Mor-Avi V, et al. Recommendations for cardiac chamber quantification by echocardiography in adults: an update from the American society of echocardiography and the European association of cardiovascular Imaging. Eur Heart J Cardiovasc Imaging 2015;16:233–70.

Valvular Heart Failure due to Tricuspid Regurgitation

Surgical and Transcatheter Management Options

Mark A. Lebehn, MD, Rebecca T. Hahn, MD*

KEYWORDS

- Tricuspid regurgitation • Transcatheter tricuspid valve devices • Heart failure
- Tricuspid valve surgery • Echocardiography

KEY POINTS

- There is an independent association of mortality with higher grades of tricuspid regurgitation severity.
- A new classification of tricuspid regurgitation etiology is derived from a more comprehensive understanding of tricuspid valve and right heart anatomy and physiology.
- Although tricuspid valve repair at the time of left heart surgery is well accepted, isolated tricuspid valve surgery is associated with high in-hospital mortality.
- Multiple transcatheter device therapies are currently under investigation to give high and prohibitive surgical risk patients treatment options beyond medical therapy.

 Video content accompanies this article at http://www.heartfailure.theclinics.com

INTRODUCTION

Tricuspid regurgitation (TR) is very common and affects 4% of individuals aged 75 years or older.[1] In the Framingham Offspring Study, mild or greater TR was found in 14.8% of men and 18.4% of women,[2] and by epidemiological data, 1.6 million US residents have moderate or greater TR.[3] Multiple studies show an independent association of mortality with higher grades of TR severity,[4–6] with even mild TR associated with worse survival and recurrent heart failure (HF) hospitalizations.[6] The presence of clinically significant TR, alone or with HF, significantly increased health-care utilization and expenditures.[7,8] Despite the high prevalence, 90% of patients with clinically significant TR historically have not been offered surgical treatment[3] in part due to the lack to level 1 recommendations in management guidelines[9,10] as well as the underdiagnosis of the disease in the setting of nonspecific symptoms and diagnostic challenges.[11] This results in delayed diagnosis after the development of hepatic and renal dysfunction, associated drivers of the high (8%–10%) associated surgical mortality.[12,13] Topilsky and colleagues found that in the follow-up of 417 community patients with moderate or greater TR followed from 1990 to 2000, only 2.6% of patients had tricuspid valve (TV) surgery during follow-up.[1] Prevalent risk factors for progression of TR have been associated with TR including: age, female sex, HF, cardiac implantable electronic device (CIED), atrial fibrillation (AF), left-sided heart disease including left atrial enlargement, elevated pulmonary artery pressures (PAP), and left-sided valvular disease.[2,14,15] Up to 50% of patients with severe mitral regurgitation and 25% with

Department of Medicine, Columbia University Medical Center/NY Presbyterian Hospital, New York, USA
* Corresponding author. Columbia University Irving Medical Center, New York-Presbyterian Hospital, 177 Fort Washington Avenue, New York, NY 10032.
E-mail address: rth2@columbia.edu

Heart Failure Clin 19 (2023) 329–343
https://doi.org/10.1016/j.hfc.2023.02.003
1551-7136/23/© 2023 Elsevier Inc. All rights reserved.

heartfailure.theclinics.com

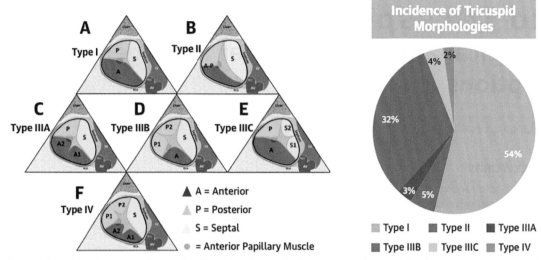

Fig. 1. Tricuspid valve nomenclature classification scheme. (*Left*) A proposed tricuspid valve nomenclature classification scheme is shown. The anterior papillary muscle is indicated as a blue circle and defines the separation of the anterior and posterior leaflets. (*A*) Type 1: 3-leaflet configuration. (*B*) Type II: 2-leaflet configuration. (*C–E*) Type III: 4-leaflet configurations. (*F*) Type IV: 5-leaflet configuration. (*Right*) Incidence of each morphology in the present study of 579 patients. A, anterior leaflet; AV, aortic valve; LV, left ventricle; NCC, noncoronary cusp; P, posterior leaflet; RCC, right coronary cusp; S, septal leaflet. (*From* Hahn RT, Weckbach LT, Noack T, et al. Proposal for a Standard Echocardiographic Tricuspid Valve Nomenclature. *JACC Cardiovasc Imaging*. Jul 2021;14(7):1299-1305.)

severe aortic stenosis develop moderate or greater TR. Following surgical or transcatheter treatment of left-sided valvular disease, persistent or worsening TR is associated with poor outcomes.[16–19] Limited recommendations for medical management and high in-hospital mortality associated with isolated TV surgery, has led to the rapid development of transcatheter devices to address this under treated population. Which patients are appropriate for medical, surgical or transcatheter therapies, and whether these therapies will improve outcomes, is the focus of multiple ongoing clinical trials and registries.

TRICUSPID VALVE ANATOMY

The TV is the largest valve with the most complex structure. The structure of the TV is composed of the leaflets, annulus, papillary muscles, and chordae. The fibrous tricuspid annulus is nonplanar and triangular or ovoid in shape.[11,20–22] The annulus is dynamic in size with a 29.6% ± 5.5% change in area throughout the cardiac cycle[23] and increases in area from end-systole to end-diastole. The normal annular circumference and area in healthy subjects are 12 ± 1 cm and 11 ± 2 cm.[22] Normal TV orifice area is between 7 and 9 cm with a transvalvular mean gradient less than 2 mm Hg with peak diastolic velocities less than 1 m/s.[22] The fibrous cardiac skeleton fixes the septal annulus, and because annular dilation

occurs, it does so in the posterolateral annular direction. With annular dilation, the annulus becomes more planar and circular. Mechanistically TR related to isolated atrial and annular dilatation, compared with TR in the setting of right ventricular (RV) remodeling, lead to differences in annular and ventricular size and shape, as well as leaflet tethering.

With the development of percutaneous therapies for the TV, there has been additional attention being paid into the variants of normal anatomy of the TV leaflets. Traditional teaching has been that the TV is composed of 3 leaflets including the anterior, posterior, and septal leaflets,[24] and with respect to attitudinal position are septal, anterosuperior, and inferior.[25] The anterior and septal leaflets are usually the longest circumferentially resulting with the anteroseptal commissure being the longest.[11] In regards to the number leaflets, studies have shown variable number of leaflets[26–28] with 3 leaflets found in 53.9%, 2 leaflets in 4.5%, 4 leaflets in 38.5%, and greater than 4 leaflets in 2.4% (**Fig. 1**).[28] The proposed naming system for the variants of leaflets uses the position of the anterior papillary muscle in labeling supernumerary leaflets beyond the customary 3 leaflet morphology.[28] Identification of the leaflets can benefit from the use of both 2D and 3D ultrasound imaging with and without color. This is of clinical importance in transcatheter edge-to-edge leaflet repair planning for device positioning.

There can be significant variability in the associated papillary muscles that include the anterior, posterior, and septal papillary muscles (attitudinal nomenclature-anterior, inferior, medial).[29] The anterior papillary muscle is useful in identification and naming of leaflets because it sends chordal attachments to both the posterior and anterior leaflets. The anterior papillary can be identified by its origin from the anterior/lateral wall of the right ventricle in the area of the trabeculations, which incorporates the moderator band.[11] Dilatation of the midright ventricle in response to pressure or volume overload, may result in the displacement of the papillary muscles and tethering of the TV leaflets.[30] In addition to primary and secondary chordae as seen with the mitral valve, the TV also has tertiary chordae, which attach directly to the septum.[25] Changes in the morphology or position of the interventricular septum may also result in tethering of the leaflets.[31]

ETIOLOGIES OF TRICUSPID REGURGITATION

The etiology of TR was historically classified into either primary (leaflet pathologic condition) or secondary (nonleaflet pathologic condition) pathologic conditions; however, a more recent expanded classification system has now been adopted (**Table 1**).[32,33] Etiologies of primary TR include rheumatic heart disease, infective endocarditis, congenital disease, myxomatous disease, carcinoid syndrome, thoracic trauma, iatrogenic valve injury, autoimmune disease, and drug induced[9,10] (Video 1). The most common form of TR is due to secondary TR (~80% secondary vs 10%–15% primary)[11] with 2 main subtypes (Video 2). Atrial secondary TR is a diagnosis of exclusion, defined by the absence of any leaflet abnormality, left ventricular (LV) dysfunction (ejection fraction <60%), left-sided valve disease, pulmonary hypertension (pulmonary artery [PA] systolic pressure >50 mm Hg)[34] or CIED, and supported by the clinical history of the patient with evidence of longstanding or permanent AF or HF with preserved ejection fraction. Leaflet mal-coaptation is the result of right atrial annular dilation with leaflets closing at or near the annular plane. Ventricular secondary TR results from leaflet tethering in the setting of ventricular dilatation and/or dysfunction often secondary to pulmonary hypertension or left-sided heart disease.[35] CIED-related TR is now a separate etiology of TR given the multifactorial pathophysiology sharing features of both primary and secondary TR in the presence of a lead. TR resulting from direct interaction of the CIED with leaflets or subvalvular apparatus is considered primary CIED-related TR (Video 3), whereas TR due to other secondary etiologies or

pacing related remodeling is considered incidental CIED-related TR. Multiple studies have found on follow-up a 21.2% to 38% prevalence of clinically significant lead-induced TR developing in patients with CIED devices.[36–38] A recent meta-analysis of 37 studies with 8144 patients, the pooled incidence of TR deterioration of at least one grade was 25.1%.[39] Lead interference (odds ratio [OR], 8.704; 95% confidence interval [CI], 4.450–17.028; $Z = 6.32$; $P < .001$) and pacemaker (vs implantable cardiac defibrillator) implantation time (OR, 1.153; 95% CI, 1.082–1.229; $Z = 4.37$; $P < .001$) were risk factors for worsening TR. All-cause mortality (>1 year after pacemaker implantation) was higher in patients with TR deterioration (hazard ratio, 1.598; 95% CI, 1.275–2.002; $Z = 4.07$; $P < .01$; $I^2 = 0\%$).

INDICATIONS FOR TREATMENT

Both the 2020 AHA/ACC and 2021 ESC/EACTS guidelines for valvular heart disease[9,10] recommend referral to a Heart Valve Center with a multidisciplinary Heart Team, which will comprehensively evaluate patient-specific, anatomic, and hemodynamic factors to optimize HF management and select the best patient-specific surgical or transcatheter option for treatment (**Fig. 2**).

In the 2020 AHA/ACC Valvular Heart Disease Guideline,[9] medical management for TR includes diuretics for right-sided HF signs and symptoms. Medical management is also recommended for therapies to treat the underlying cause of secondary TR (eg, pulmonary vasodilators, guideline-directed medical therapy for HF, or rhythm control for AF). A class I recommendation for TV surgery is given for patients undergoing left-sided valve surgery with severe TR (Stages C and D) and with progressive TR with signs and symptoms of right-sided HF, or with tricuspid annular dilation greater than 4.0 cm (Class IIA). Isolated TV surgery can be considered to reduce symptoms and recurrent hospitalizations in the setting of right-sided HF and severe primary TR (Class IIA) or in patients with secondary TR due to annular dilation who are poorly responsive to medical management (Class IIA). TV surgery can also be considered in asymptomatic patients with severe primary TR with progressive RV dilation or dysfunction (Class IIB) or can be considered with signs and symptoms of right-sided HF and severe TR who have undergone earlier left-sided valve surgery in the absence of severe pulmonary hypertension or severe RV dysfunction (Class IIB). In the absence of any US Food and Drug Administration approved transcatheter device, there are no guideline recommendations for this management strategy;

Table 1
New classification of tricuspid regurgitation

Etiology		Leaflet Structure	Pathophysiology	Etiology	Imaging
Secondary (Functional)					
A. Atrial	Normal		RA enlargement and dysfunction leading to significant isolated annulus dilation; RV often normal	Carpentier I: Atrial fibrillation/flutter Age Heart failure with preserved ejection fraction	Marked *TV annulus dilation* is the dominant mechanism TV leaflet tethering is absent or minimal (except for late stages with secondary RV dysfunction) TV leaflet mobility is typically normal (Carpentier type I) RA is significantly dilated RV volume is typically normal (except for late stages) *RV basal diameter may appear abnormal due to the conical RV shape*
B. Ventricular	Normal		RV enlargement and/or dysfunction leading to significant leaflet tethering and annulus dilation	Carpentier IIIB: Left-sided ventricular or valvular disease Pulmonary hypertension RV cardiomyopathy RV infarction	Marked *TV leaflet tethering* is the dominant mechanism TV leaflet mobility is typically restricted in systole (Carpentier type IIIB) TV annulus, RV and RA are dilated ± dysfunctional
CIED-related (primary vs incidental)	Normal/abnormal		Leaflet impingement Leaflet/chordal entanglement Leaflet adherence Leaflet laceration/perforation Leaflet avulsion (after lead extraction)	Pacemaker Implantable cardiac defibrillator (ICD) Cardiac resynchronization therapy (CRT)	*TV leaflet structural abnormalities* may be present TV leaflet mobility is variable (all Carpentier types) TV annulus, RV and RA are typically dilated (except for acute TR)

| Primary (Organic) | Abnormal | Lack of leaflet coaptation due to intrinsic changes leading to restricted or excessive leaflet mobility or leaflet perforation | Carpentier I: Congenital Endocarditis Carpentier II: Myxomatous disease Traumatic Postbiopsy Carpentier IIIA: Carcinoid Rheumatic Radiotherapy tumors* | *TV leaflet structural abnormalities* characteristic for each primary etiology are the dominant mechanisms TV leaflet mobility is variable (all Carpentier types) TV annulus, RV and RA are typically dilated (except for acute TR) |

Abbreviations: CIED, cardiac implantable electronic device; CRT, cardiac resynchronization therapy; ICD, implantable cardiac defibrillator; RA, right atrium; RV, right ventricle; TR, tricuspid regurgitation; TV, tricuspid valve.

* RV basal diameter may appear abnormal due to the conical RV shape.

From Praz F, Muraru D, Kreidel F, et al. Transcatheter treatment for tricuspid valve disease. *EuroIntervention*. 2021;17(10):791-808.

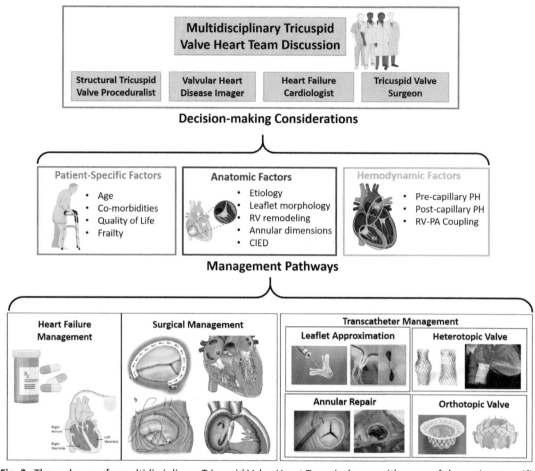

Fig. 2. The make-up of a multidisciplinary Tricuspid Valve Heart Team is shown with some of the patient-specific, anatomic, and hemodynamic factors that are incorporated into the decision-making for appropriate heart failure management, which may be augmented with surgical or transcatheter therapies.

however, 3 randomized trials are currently enrolling.

The recommendations of the European Society of Cardiology/European Association of Cardiothoracic Surgeons[10] differ slightly from the ACC/AHA guidelines. Medical therapy does not receive a clear class of recommendation; however, the guidelines states that (1) diuretics are useful in the presence of right-sided HF, and the addition of an aldosterone antagonist may be considered; (2) dedicated treatment of pulmonary hypertension is indicated in specific cases; (3) although data are limited, rhythm control may help to decrease TR and contain annular dilatation in patients with chronic AF; and (4) in the absence of advanced RV dysfunction or severe pulmonary hypertension, none of the above-mentioned therapies should delay the referral for surgery or transcatheter therapy. Four devices have received Conformité Européenne (CE) *conformité européenne* Mark for treatment of TR, thus the guidelines give a Class IIB recommendation for transcatheter TV intervention of symptomatic secondary severe TR may be considered in inoperable patients at a Heart Valve Center with expertise in the treatment of TV disease.

RIGHT HEART ASSESSMENT

In patients with significant TR, RV remodeling due to both dilatation and dysfunction should be assessed.[40] A thorough evaluation of RV size and function is critical and guidelines exist for the echocardiographic assessment of the right heart.[41,42] TR leads to a viscous cycle of remodeling of tissue, RV shape, and function.[32] A multimodality imaging approach can be taken with use of 2D/3D echocardiography, cardiac computed tomography, and cardiac MRI (CMR). The principal imaging modality has been assessment by echocardiography. Multiple different methods can be used to assess RV function including tricuspid annular plane systolic excursion (TAPSE), tissue-Doppler systolic annular velocity, fractional area change, RV ejection fraction by 3D, and RV free wall or global longitudinal strain. Contractile reserve can be assessed by stress echocardiography or CMR and RV tissue remodeling can be assessed for with CMR T1 and T2 mapping, evaluating for any evidence of late gadolinium enhancement and calculation of extracellular volume.

Measurements of RV function have important prognostic value in patients with TR.[40,43,44] Indexing RV contractility to afterload, or RV-PA coupling, describes a normal physiologic state where mechanical stroke work is transferred efficiently to the pulmonary circuit and RV contractility can increase when afterload increases. Echocardiographic measures of RV function can thus be indexed to estimates of PAP to assess RV-PA coupling. Doppler estimates of systolic PAP (sPAP) may underestimate invasive measurements, particularly in the setting of greater TR severity, worse LV and RV function, and the V-wave cutoff sign on spectral Doppler[45]; however, despite this known limitation, TAPSE/sPAP in patients with severe secondary TR was shown to be independently associated with all-cause mortality.[46] Baseline and changes in RV-PA coupling are predictors of outcomes following transcatheter TV interventions.[47] Given the different outcomes associated with precapillary and postcapillary pulmonary hypertension in the setting of significant TR,[48] a right heart catheterization is recommended to differentiate these entities.[49]

Three-dimensional transthoracic echocardiography (TTE) compares favorably with CMR for quantitation of volumes[50] and can be used to quantify RV and atrial volumes, as well as TV tenting volume and annular area.[30] Recent studies have suggested by an RV ejection fraction of 45% or less by either CMR[51] or 3D TTE[52] is predictive of poor outcomes following transcatheter TV repair.

SURGICAL APPROACHES

Isolated TV surgery is associated with an in-hospital mortality of 8% to 10%.[12,13] In a recent study in which a dedicated risk score model was developed to predict the outcome of patients after isolated TV surgery for severe TR using 8 parameters: age 70 years or older (1 point), New York Heart Association Class III-IV (1 point), right-sided HF signs (2 points), daily dose of furosemide 125 mg or greater (2 points), glomerular filtration rate less than 30 mL/min (2 points), elevated bilirubin (2 points), LV ejection fraction less than 60% (1 point), and moderate/severe RV dysfunction (1 point). Isolated tricuspid surgery, when

performed in patients without comorbidities, preserved RV function, and no organ failure (ie, a risk score of ≤3), is associated with an in-hospital mortality of 5% or less.[53] In low-risk patients, surgery remains the gold standard treatment of functional TR.[34,54]

The choice among the different surgical and interventional options available to treat TR[55–57] should be driven by the underlying mechanism of TR, the patient conditions, and the cause of the disease. The anatomo-functional assessment of the TV becomes of primary importance to choose between replacement and repair. In patients with anatomy suitable for repair, the fine details of anatomy and function of the valve components can influence the repair strategy and the techniques used.

There are multiple surgical TV repair techniques including edge-to-edge suture (eg, Clover technique), suture obliterating repair (eg, Kay repair), annuloplasty, neo-chords, and leaflet augmentation. Tricuspid annuloplasty can be accomplished with suture-only (eg, De Vega) techniques versus with a ring, band, or pericardial strip. Annuloplasty rings and bands come in various designs with rigid, semirigid, flexible, and biodegradable designs. Risk factors for recurrent TR and failure of repair include: severity of preoperative TR, pulmonary hypertension, RV postoperative function, TV annular diameter, leaflet tethering and RV: dysfunction, enlargement, sphericity, and width.[58–66] Despite numerous available surgical repair techniques to address functional TR, moderate or greater TR has been found in 15% to 20% of patients within the first year and 30% to 70% at 5 years.[58]

When replacement is thought to be a better option than repair with annuloplasty (eg, endocarditis, rheumatic, carcinoid disease, leaflet tethering, severe annular dilation) bioprosthetic valve replacement is the principle form of replacement over mechanical valves due to risk of thrombosis and requirement of warfarin therapy. In addition, the use of an atrioventricular homografts has been described in individual patients and case series.[67] Predictors of worsening TR after annuloplasty for secondary TR include higher grade of preoperative TR, poor LV function, permanent pacemaker, and nonring annuloplasty repair technique.[68] Current surgical techniques also include minimally invasive surgery, which may be of benefit compared with median sternotomy for high-risk patients although randomized controlled trials comparing these approaches is lacking.[69]

TRANSCATHETER APPROACHES

Transcatheter TV intervention treatment options can be broadly be classified into the following groups: transcatheter edge-to-edge repair (TEER), direct annuloplasty, transcatheter TV implantation, and heterotopic caval valve implantation (**Fig. 3**).[32] Favorable to unfavorable anatomical features have been shown to assist with device choice (**Table 2**)[32] and proposed algorithms for device choice consider the cause, leaflet pathologic condition, coaptation gaps of the leaflets, and stage of presentation. However, because we learn more about the complexities of each class of device, the decision-making process is less of a simple algorithm but rather a multiparametric consideration that required thoughtful input from an experienced TV Heart Team (**Fig. 4**). Intraprocedural imaging may include TTE, transesophageal echocardiography, intracardiac echocardiography, fluoroscopy, and fusion imaging.

Edge-to-edge repair: TV TEER uses leaflet approximation technology initially developed for the mitral valve.[70–72] The MitraClip (Abbott Vascular, Santa Clara, CA, USA), TriClip (Abbott Vascular, Santa Clara, CA, USA), and PASCAL systems (Edwards Lifesciences, Irvine, CA, USA) have both been shown to have high procedural success, acceptable safety, and significant clinical improvement.[70–75] These devices have multiple implant sizes and widths, and the ability for independent leaflet grasping to replicate in concept the surgical Alfieri stich repair technique. The TRILUMINATE trial with the use of the TriClip™ in the treatment of 85 patients with symptomatic moderate or greater TR who were high risk for surgery showed a durable 1-year result with 87% having 1+ or greater sustained reduction in TR grade and 70% having moderate or less TR at 1 year.[74] This trial also demonstrated the importance of monitoring of disease progression and early treatment as baseline TR was shown as the only significant predictor of achieving moderate or less TR at 1-year postrepair. Massive and torrential TR before repair was less likely to achieve moderate or less TR at follow-up compared with starting with severe TR at the time of repair. TV-TEER has shown to lead to improvements in HF symptoms, 6-minute walk distance, and reductions in hospitalizations and mortality.[72,74,76] The CLASP TR trial 1-year results, with the use of the PASCAL system, showed 88% of patients with greater than 1-grade reduction in TR, 86% of patients with moderate or less TR at 1 year, and improvements in NYHA class, 6MWD

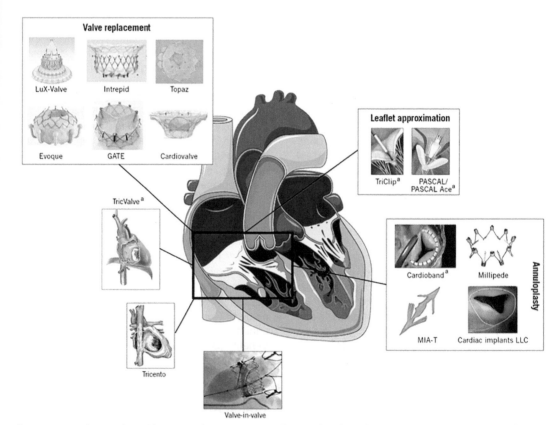

Fig. 3. Transcatheter tricuspid systems that are approved or under clinical evaluation. [a]With CE approval. (*From* Praz F, Muraru D, Kreidel F, et al. Transcatheter treatment for tricuspid valve disease. *EuroIntervention.* 2021;17(10):791-808.

Table 2
Anatomic criteria for device selection

Strategy	Favorable Anatomy	Feasible Anatomy	Unfavorable Anatomy
Leaflet approximation	• Small septolateral gap ≤7 mm • Anteroseptal jet location • Confined prolapse or flail • Trileaflet morphology	• Septolateral gap >7 but <8.5 mm • Posteroseptal jet location • Nontrileaflet morphology • Incidental CIED (ie, without leaflet impingement)	• Large septolateral gap >8.5 mm • Leaflet thickening/shortening (rheumatic, carcinoid)/perforation • Dense chordae with marked leaflet tethering • Anteroposterior jet location • Poor echocardiographic leaflet visualization • CIED leaflet impingement • Unfavorable device angle of approach
Annuloplasty	• Annular dilatation as primary mechanism of TR • Mild tethering (tenting height <0.76 cm, tenting area <1.63 cm2, tenting volume [3D] <2.3 mL) • Central jet location • Sufficient landing zone for anchoring	• Moderate tethering (tethering height ≥0.76 cm but <1.0 cm, tenting area >1.63 but <2.5 cm², tenting volume [3D] ≥2.3 mL but ≤3.5 mL) • Incidental CIED (ie, without leaflet impingement)	• Excessive annular dilatation (exceeding device size) • Severe tethering (tethering height >1.0 cm, tenting volume >3.5 mL) Poor echocardiographic annular visualization • Annular proximity of RCA • CIED leaflet impingement
Orthotopic valve implantation	• Previous surgical repair or bioprosthetic valve replacement • Leaflet thickening/shortening (rheumatic, carcinoid) • Incidental CIED (ie, without leaflet impingement) • Any leaflet morphology	• Large gap >9 mm • CIED leaflet impingement	• Excessive annular dilatation (exceeding device size) • Unfavorable device angle of approach • Severe right ventricular dysfunction
Heterotopic valve implantation	• Appropriate caval diameters (and intercaval distance) • No option for direct valve treatment		• Proximity of the RA to the orifice of the liver veins • Severely increased pulmonary artery and RA pressures

From Praz F, Muraru D, Kreidel F, et al. Transcatheter treatment for tricuspid valve disease. *EuroIntervention.* 2021;17(10):791-808.

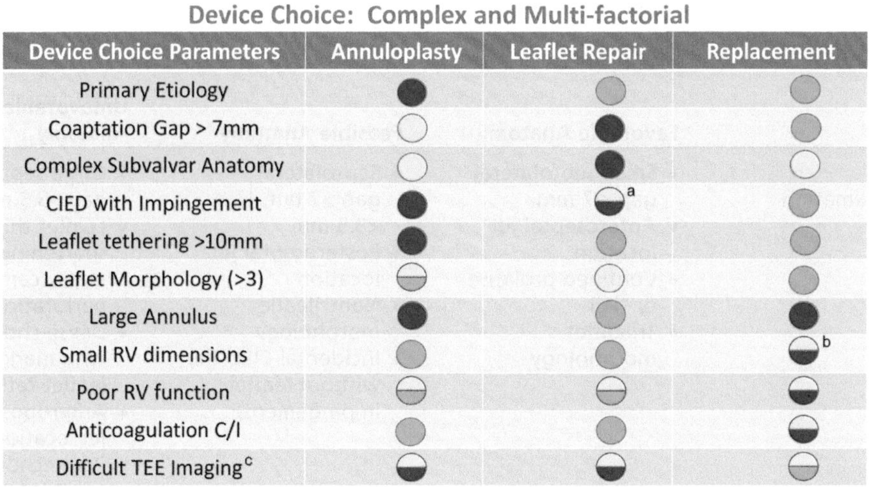

Device Choice: Complex and Multi-factorial

Device Choice Parameters	Annuloplasty	Leaflet Repair	Replacement
Primary Etiology	●	◔	◔
Coaptation Gap > 7mm	○	●	○
Complex Subvalvar Anatomy	○	●	○
CIED with Impingement	●	◐[a]	○
Leaflet tethering >10mm	●	○	◔
Leaflet Morphology (>3)	⊖	○	◔
Large Annulus	●	○	●
Small RV dimensions	◔	○	◐[b]
Poor RV function	⊖	⊖	⊖
Anticoagulation C/I	◔	◔	⊖
Difficult TEE Imaging[c]	⊖	◐	⊖

Fig. 4. Shown are the anatomic, patient-specific, and imaging factors that are considered in the decision-making for either repair with annuloplasty or repair versus replacement. [a]Dependent on location of TR, [b]Dependent on Device, [c]ICE Imaging may be useful.

and improvement in health status by KCCQ scores (presented by Dr Adan Greenbaum at American College of Cardiology annual Congress in 2022). As an additional alternative the novel DragonFly device (Valgen Medical, Hong Kong, China), which was recently successfully used to repair the mitral valve,[77] is also under investigation for use on the TV.

Another device that addresses leaflet coaptation is the Mistral (Mitralix, Yok'neam, Israel) device. This novel device uses a spiral shaped nitinol wire to grasp the chordae tendineae that are attached to different adjacent leaflets, creating a "bouquet" of the chordae and thus approximating the leaflets. This theoretically improves leaflet coaptation and modifies the geometry of the RV. The first-in-human experience of 7 implants showed no 30-day adverse events, with reduction of TR (~50–60%) and improvement of RV function and exercise capacity.[78]

Annuloplasty: Multiple direct and indirect annuloplasty systems have been under development to address annular dilation in functional TR. The Cardioband Tricuspid System (Edwards Lifescience, Irvine, CA) implant is composed of a polyester sleeve with radiopaque markers mounted on a delivery system with 17 stainless steel anchors. The Cardioband delivery system is delivered via a transfemoral venous approach and consists of an implant delivery system (IDS) and 24F steerable sheath. The IDS is steered to the antero-septal commissure and the anchors are sequentially deployed along the atrial surface of the annulus to the postero-septal commissure. Cinching of the device and sizing is accomplished with a contraction wire with the use of a size adjustment tool. The TRI-REPAIR study evaluated the safety and efficacy of the Cardioband

device in 30 prohibitive risk patients with moderate-to-severe TR and annular dilation. Published data at 2-year follow-up showed a sustained repair with a significant reduction in TR due to reduced annular dimension (average 16% reduction in septolateral diameter at 2 years), and 72% of patients with moderate or less TR.[79]

Other annuloplasty devices in clinical trials include the C1 Percutaneous Ring Annuloplasty system, and the DaVingi System. The first-in-human experience with the DaVingi TR system reported successful reduction in TR from massive to mild, during the follow-up period.[80]

Transcatheter tricuspid valve replacement (TTVR): Although transcatheter TV replacement remains investigational in the United States, the field of potential devices is already broad. There has been an evolution from surgical thoracotomy or transjugular approach to a transfemoral approach. Current valves being evaluated for transfemoral TTVR include the EVOQUE (Edwards Lifesciences, Irvine, California), Intrepid (Medtronic PLC, Minneapolis, MN), CardioValve (Cardiovalve Ltd., Or Yehuda, Israel), and Topaz (TRiCares, Aschheim, Munich, Germany). The LuX-Valve (Jencare Biotechnology Co., Ningbo, China) is a transcatheter valve with the current generation of the valve using a transjugular approach. In the future device choice may be based on characteristics including annular size, approach angle of the inferior vena cava, leaflet pathologic condition being addressed and femoral access. The largest clinical experience is with the EVOQUE system from the outcomes from the compassionate use experience and from the 30-day results of the TRISCEND trial (NCT04221490). In the compassionate use experience with 27 inoperable or high-risk patients, 1-year follow-up results showed a mortality of 7%, 70% of patients were NYHA functional class I/II, and 96% of patients had 2+ or less TR.[81] In the follow-up from 30-days to 1-year HF hospitalizations were reported in only 2 patients. In the TRISCEND study of 56 patients with moderate or greater TR, there was a procedural success rate of 92.9% with mild or less TR found in 98% of patients at 30-days.[82] The TRISCEND Pivotal trial (NCT04482062) is currently enrolling. Individual patient experiences have been reported with the Intrepid, CardioValve, and Topaz valves, with studies to evaluate the CardioValve (NCT04100720) and Topaz (NCT05126030) valves planned. Twelve-month results in the first-in-human experience with the LuX-Valve were presented at TVT Structural Heart Summit in June, 2022 and showed 100% procedural success rate with a TR reduction to mild or less TR in 85.2% of patients and a high rate of persistent improvement of symptoms and survival at 1 year.[83] Ongoing trials include the LuX-Valve TRAVEL TRIAL (NCT04436653), TRAVEL II TRIAL (NCT05194423), and second-generation LuX-Valve Plus delivered through transjugular access (NCT 05436028).

Heterotopic bicaval stenting: In high risk or inoperable patients with anatomy unsuitable for TTVR or TEER, heterotopic caval implantation may be considered to alleviate symptoms and upstream deleterious effects of TR. The TRICENTO THV (New Valve Technology, Hechingen, Germany) is a custom-made covered nitinol stent, spanning and thus anchored in both cavae, with a lateral porcine bicuspid valve element. Early clinical experience with 21 high-risk patients showed 100% technical success with symptomatic improvement (65% of patients improved NYHA class III/IV symptoms to class I/II).[84] The TricValve System (P + F Products + Features, Vienna, Austria) consists of 2 (inferior vena cava and superior vena cava specific) self-expanding nitinol stents, which hold bovine pericardial leaflets. In the TRICUS EURO study evaluating the TricValve in 35 high-risk patients on optimal medical therapy, a high procedural success rate was found (94%), and at 6 months follow-up 79.4% of patients reported NYHA class I or II symptoms, all-cause mortality was 8.5%, and HF hospitalization was only 20%.[85]

POSTPROCEDURAL MANAGEMENT

Patients' postprocedure requires close monitoring of volume status may require titration of diuretics. Depending on the device, antiplatelet therapy versus oral anticoagulation with warfarin may be required. Repeat imaging should be obtained to evaluate for success of repair and to evaluate for RV reverse remodeling over time. Routine follow-up should be scheduled in the treating Heart Valve Center. If an investigational device is used, depending on the study follow-up protocol, testing may include cardiac markers, renal and liver function testing, TTE, a 6-minute walk test, and a quality-of-life questionnaire. Recommendations in regards to infective endocarditis prophylaxis follow the recommendations of the 2020 ACC/AHA Guideline for the Management of Patients with Valvular Heart Disease.[86]

SUMMARY

Appropriate diagnosis and treatment of patients with TR requires an understanding of the complex structure of the TV anatomy and surrounding structures. Care of patients with symptomatic severe TR requires a multidisciplinary team approach with involvement of the patient's general cardiologist, structural interventional cardiologist, structural imaging cardiologist, and HF specialists. To accurately define the cause, severity, determine appropriate therapy, intraprocedural guidance, and guide follow-up management, a multimodality imaging approach is beneficial (eg, TTE, cardiac CT, and CMR). With these aspects in mind all patients benefit from an early referral to a Comprehensive Valve Center[9] with a TV Heart Team for the coordination of the specialized care and imaging required. It is currently an exciting time for those caring for patients with TV regurgitation, as transcatheter therapeutic treatment options are rapidly expanding to supplement current surgical treatments.

CLINICS CARE POINTS

- There is an independent association of mortality with higher grades of TR severity.
- A new classification of TR etiology is derived from a more comprehensive understanding of TV anatomy and physiology, as well as right heart remodeling and function.
- Although TV repair at the time of left heart surgery is well accepted, isolated TV surgery is associated with high in-hospital mortality.
- Multiple transcatheter device therapies are currently under investigation to give high and prohibitive surgical risk patients treatment options beyond medical therapy.

DISCLOSURE

Dr R.T. Hahn reports speaker fees from Abbott Vascular, Baylis Medical, and Edwards Lifesciences; institutional consulting for Abbott Structural, Edwards Lifesciences, Medtronic; equity with Navigate; and is Chief Scientific Officer for the Echocardiography Core Laboratory at the Cardiovascular Research Foundation for multiple industry-sponsored trials, for which she receives no direct industry compensation.

SUPPLEMENTARY DATA

Supplementary data related to this article can be found online at https://doi.org/10.1016/j.hfc.2023.02.003.

REFERENCES

1. Topilsky Y, Maltais S, Medina Inojosa J, et al. Burden of Tricuspid Regurgitation in Patients Diagnosed in the Community Setting. JACC Cardiovasc Imaging 2019;12(3):433–42.
2. Singh JP, Evans JC, Levy D, et al. Prevalence and clinical determinants of mitral, tricuspid, and aortic regurgitation (the Framingham Heart Study). Am J Cardiol 1999;83(6):897–902.
3. Enriquez-Sarano M, Messika-Zeitoun D, Topilsky Y, et al. Tricuspid regurgitation is a public health crisis. Prog Cardiovasc Dis 2019;62(6):447–51.
4. Chorin E, Rozenbaum Z, Topilsky Y, et al. Tricuspid regurgitation and long-term clinical outcomes. European Heart Journal Cardiovascular IMAGING 2020; 21(2):157–65.
5. Benfari G, Antoine C, Miller WL, et al. Excess Mortality Associated With Functional Tricuspid Regurgitation Complicating Heart Failure With Reduced Ejection Fraction. Circulation 2019;140(3): 196–206.
6. Offen S, Playford D, Strange G, et al. Adverse Prognostic Impact of Even Mild or Moderate Tricuspid Regurgitation: Insights from the National Echocardiography Database of Australia. J Am Soc Echocardiogr 2022;35(8):810–7.
7. Cork DP, McCullough PA, Mehta HS, et al. The economic impact of clinically significant tricuspid regurgitation in a large, administrative claims database. J Med Econ 2020;23(5):521–8.
8. Barker CM, Cork DP, McCullough PA, et al. Healthcare utilization in clinically significant tricuspid regurgitation patients with and without heart failure. J Comp Eff Res 2021;10(1):29–37.
9. Otto CM, Nishimura RA, Bonow RO, et al. 2020 ACC/AHA Guideline for the Management of Patients With Valvular Heart Disease: A Report of the American College of Cardiology/American Heart Association Joint Committee on Clinical Practice Guidelines. J Am Coll Cardiol 2021;77(4):e25–197.
10. Vahanian A, Beyersdorf F, Praz F, et al. 2021 ESC/EACTS Guidelines for the management of valvular heart disease. Eur Heart J 2022;43(7):561–632.
11. Hahn RT, Badano LP, Bartko PE, et al. Tricuspid regurgitation: recent advances in understanding pathophysiology, severity grading and outcome. European Heart Journal Cardiovascular Imaging 2022; 23(7):913–29.
12. LaPar DJ, Likosky DS, Zhang M, et al. Development of a Risk Prediction Model and Clinical Risk Score for Isolated Tricuspid Valve Surgery. Ann Thorac Surg 2018;106(1):129–36.
13. Vassileva CM, Shabosky J, Boley T, et al. Tricuspid valve surgery: the past 10 years from the Nationwide Inpatient Sample (NIS) database. J Thorac Cardiovasc Surg 2012;143(5):1043–9.
14. Topilsky Y, Nkomo VT, Vatury O, et al. Clinical outcome of isolated tricuspid regurgitation. JACC Cardiovasc Imaging 2014;7(12):1185–94.
15. Mutlak D, Khalil J, Lessick J, et al. Risk Factors for the Development of Functional Tricuspid Regurgitation and Their Population-Attributable Fractions. JACC Cardiovasc Imaging 2020;13(8):1643–51.
16. Cremer PC, Wang TKM, Rodriguez LL, et al. Incidence and Clinical Significance of Worsening Tricuspid Regurgitation Following Surgical or Transcatheter Aortic Valve Replacement: Analysis From the PARTNER IIA Trial. Circ Cardiovasc Interv 2021;14(8):e010437.
17. Truong VT, Ngo TNM, Mazur J, et al. Right ventricular dysfunction and tricuspid regurgitation in functional mitral regurgitation. ESC heart failure 2021; 8(6):4988–96.
18. Hahn RT, Asch F, Weissman NJ, et al. Impact of Tricuspid Regurgitation on Clinical Outcomes: The COAPT Trial. J Am Coll Cardiol 2020;76(11): 1305–14.
19. Kavsur R, Iliadis C, Spieker M, et al. Predictors and prognostic relevance of tricuspid alterations in patients undergoing transcatheter edge-to-edge mitral valve repair. EuroIntervention 2021;17(10):827–34.
20. Irwin RB, Luckie M, Khattar RS. Tricuspid regurgitation: contemporary management of a neglected valvular lesion. Postgrad Med J. Nov 2010; 86(1021):648–55.
21. Dreyfus GD, Martin RP, Chan KM, et al. Functional tricuspid regurgitation: a need to revise our understanding. J Am Coll Cardiol 2015;65(21):2331–6.
22. Hahn RT. State-of-the-Art Review of Echocardiographic Imaging in the Evaluation and Treatment of Functional Tricuspid Regurgitation. Circ Cardiovasc Imaging 2016;9(12). https://doi.org/10.1161/CIRCIMAGING.116.005332.
23. Addetia K, Muraru D, Veronesi F, et al. 3-Dimensional Echocardiographic Analysis of the Tricuspid

Annulus Provides New Insights Into Tricuspid Valve Geometry and Dynamics. JACC Cardiovasc Imaging 2019;12(3):401–12.

24. Silver MD, Lam JH, Ranganathan N, et al. Morphology of the human tricuspid valve. Circulation 1971;43(3):333–48.

25. Martinez RM, O'Leary PW, Anderson RH. Anatomy and echocardiography of the normal and abnormal tricuspid valve. Cardiol Young 2006;16(Suppl 3): 4–11.

26. Bateman MG, Quill JL, Hill AJ, et al. The clinical anatomy and pathology of the human atrioventricular valves: implications for repair or replacement. J Cardiovasc Transl Res 2013;6(2):155–65.

27. Kocak A, Govsa F, Aktas EO, et al. Structure of the human tricuspid valve leaflets and its chordae tendineae in unexpected death. A forensic autopsy study of 400 cases. Saudi Med J 2004;25(8):1051–9.

28. Hahn RT, Weckbach LT, Noack T, et al. Proposal for a Standard Echocardiographic Tricuspid Valve Nomenclature. JACC Cardiovasc Imaging 2021; 14(7):1299–305.

29. Tretter JT, Sarwark AE, Anderson RH, et al. Assessment of the anatomical variation to be found in the normal tricuspid valve. Clin Anat 2016;29(3): 399–407.

30. Muraru D, Addetia K, Guta AC, et al. Right atrial volume is a major determinant of tricuspid annulus area in functional tricuspid regurgitation: a three-dimensional echocardiographic study. Eur Heart J Cardiovasc Imaging 2021;22(6):660–9.

31. Muraru D, Hahn RT, Soliman OI, et al. 3-Dimensional Echocardiography in Imaging the Tricuspid Valve. JACC Cardiovasc Imaging 2019;12(3):500–15.

32. Praz F, Muraru D, Kreidel F, et al. Transcatheter treatment for tricuspid valve disease. EuroIntervention 2021;17(10):791–808.

33. Lancellotti P, Pibarot P, Chambers J, et al. Multi-modality imaging assessment of native valvular regurgitation: an EACVI and ESC council of valvular heart disease position paper. European heart journal cardiovascular Imaging 2022. https://doi.org/10.1093/ehjci/jeab253.

34. Otto CM, Nishimura RA, Bonow RO, et al. 2020 ACC/AHA Guideline for the Management of Patients With Valvular Heart Disease: Executive Summary: A Report of the American College of Cardiology/American Heart Association Joint Committee on Clinical Practice Guidelines. J Am Coll Cardiol 2021;77(4): 450–500.

35. Pibarot P, Messika-Zeitoun D, Ben-Yehuda O, et al. Moderate Aortic Stenosis and Heart Failure With Reduced Ejection Fraction: Can Imaging Guide Us to Therapy? JACC Cardiovasc Imaging 2019;12(1): 172–84.

36. Kim JB, Spevack DM, Tunick PA, et al. The effect of transvenous pacemaker and implantable cardioverter defibrillator lead placement on tricuspid valve function: an observational study. J Am Soc Echocardiogr 2008;21(3):284–7.

37. Hoke U, Auger D, Thijssen J, et al. Significant lead-induced tricuspid regurgitation is associated with poor prognosis at long-term follow-up. Heart 2014; 100(12):960–8.

38. Anvardeen K, Rao R, Hazra S, et al. Prevalence and Significance of Tricuspid Regurgitation Post-Endocardial Lead Placement. JACC Cardiovasc Imaging 2019;12(3):562–4.

39. Zhang XX, Wei M, Xiang R, et al. Incidence, Risk Factors, and Prognosis of Tricuspid Regurgitation After Cardiac Implantable Electronic Device Implantation: A Systematic Review and Meta-analysis. J Cardiothorac Vasc Anesth 2022;36(6):1741–55.

40. Florescu DR, Muraru D, Florescu C, et al. Right heart chambers geometry and function in patients with the atrial and the ventricular phenotypes of functional tricuspid regurgitation. European heart journal cardiovascular Imaging 2022;23(7):930–40.

41. Rudski LG, Lai WW, Afilalo J, et al. Guidelines for the echocardiographic assessment of the right heart in adults: a report from the American Society of Echocardiography endorsed by the European Association of Echocardiography, a registered branch of the European Society of Cardiology, and the Canadian Society of Echocardiography. J Am Soc Echocardiogr 2010;23(7):685–713. quiz 786-8.

42. Lang RM, Badano LP, Mor-Avi V, et al. Recommendations for cardiac chamber quantification by echocardiography in adults: an update from the American Society of Echocardiography and the European Association of Cardiovascular Imaging. Eur Heart J Cardiovasc Imaging 2015;16(3):233–70.

43. Dietz MF, Prihadi EA, van der Bijl P, et al. Prognostic Implications of Right Ventricular Remodeling and Function in Patients With Significant Secondary Tricuspid Regurgitation. Circulation 2019;140(10): 836–45.

44. Prihadi EA, van der Bijl P, Dietz M, et al. Prognostic Implications of Right Ventricular Free Wall Longitudinal Strain in Patients With Significant Functional Tricuspid Regurgitation. Circ Cardiovasc Imaging 2019;12(3):e008666.

45. Lurz P, Orban M, Besler C, et al. Clinical characteristics, diagnosis, and risk stratification of pulmonary hypertension in severe tricuspid regurgitation and implications for transcatheter tricuspid valve repair. Eur Heart J 2020;41(29):2785–95.

46. Fortuni F, Butcher SC, Dietz MF, et al. Right Ventricular-Pulmonary Arterial Coupling in Secondary Tricuspid Regurgitation. Am J Cardiol 2021; 148:138–45.

47. Brener MI, Lurz P, Hausleiter J, et al. Right Ventricular-Pulmonary Arterial Coupling and Afterload Reserve in Patients Undergoing Transcatheter

Tricuspid Valve Repair. J Am Coll Cardiol 2022; 79(5):448–61.

48. Stocker TJ, Hertell H, Orban M, et al. Cardiopulmonary Hemodynamic Profile Predicts Mortality After Transcatheter Tricuspid Valve Repair in Chronic Heart Failure. JACC Cardiovasc Interv 2021;14(1): 29–38.

49. Humbert M, Kovacs G, Hoeper MM, et al. 2022 ESC/ERS Guidelines for the diagnosis and treatment of pulmonary hypertension. Eur Heart J 2022. https://doi.org/10.1093/eurheartj/ehac237.

50. Park JB, Lee SP, Lee JH, et al. Quantification of Right Ventricular Volume and Function Using Single-Beat Three-Dimensional Echocardiography: A Validation Study with Cardiac Magnetic Resonance. J Am Soc Echocardiogr 2016;29(5):392–401.

51. Kresoja KP, Rommel KP, Lucke C, et al. Right Ventricular Contraction Patterns in Patients Undergoing Transcatheter Tricuspid Valve Repair for Severe Tricuspid Regurgitation. JACC Cardiovasc Interv 2021;14(14):1551–61.

52. Orban M, Wolff S, Braun D, et al. Right Ventricular Function in Transcatheter Edge-to-Edge Tricuspid Valve Repair. JACC (J Am Coll Cardiol): Cardiovascular Imaging 2021;14(12):2477–9.

53. Dreyfus J, Audureau E, Bohbot Y, et al. TRI-SCORE: a new risk score for in-hospital mortality prediction after isolated tricuspid valve surgery. Eur Heart J 2021. https://doi.org/10.1093/eurheartj/ehab679.

54. Vahanian A, Beyersdorf F, Praz F, et al. 2021 ESC/EACTS Guidelines for the management of valvular heart disease: Developed by the Task Force for the management of valvular heart disease of the European Society of Cardiology (ESC) and the European Association for Cardio-Thoracic Surgery (EACTS). Eur Heart J 2021. https://doi.org/10.1093/eurheartj/ehab395.

55. Rodes-Cabau J, Hahn RT, Latib A, et al. Transcatheter Therapies for Treating Tricuspid Regurgitation. J Am Coll Cardiol 2016;67(15):1829–45.

56. Taramasso M, Gavazzoni M, Pozzoli A, et al. Tricuspid Regurgitation: Predicting the Need for Intervention, Procedural Success, and Recurrence of Disease. JACC Cardiovasc Imaging 2019;12(4):605–21.

57. Taramasso M, Maisano F. Transcatheter tricuspid valve intervention: state of the art. EuroIntervention 2017;13(AA):AA40–50.

58. Maslow A, Abisse S, Parikh L, et al. Echocardiographic Predictors of Tricuspid Ring Annuloplasty Repair Failure for Functional Tricuspid Regurgitation. J Cardiothorac Vasc Anesth 2019;33(10): 2624–33.

59. Duran CM, Pomar JL, Colman T, et al. Is tricuspid valve repair necessary? J Thorac Cardiovasc Surg 1980;80(6):849–60.

60. Goldman ME, Guarino T, Fuster V, et al. The necessity for tricuspid valve repair can be determined intraoperatively by two-dimensional echocardiography. J Thorac Cardiovasc Surg 1987;94(4):542–50.

61. Matsunaga A, Duran CM. Progression of tricuspid regurgitation after repaired functional ischemic mitral regurgitation. Circulation 2005;112(9 Suppl): I453–7.

62. Fukuda S, Gillinov AM, Song JM, et al. Echocardiographic insights into atrial and ventricular mechanisms of functional tricuspid regurgitation. Am Heart J 2006;152(6):1208–14.

63. Fukuda S, Gillinov AM, McCarthy PM, et al. Echocardiographic follow-up of tricuspid annuloplasty with a new three-dimensional ring in patients with functional tricuspid regurgitation. J Am Soc Echocardiogr 2007;20(11):1236–42.

64. Fukuda S, Gillinov AM, McCarthy PM, et al. Determinants of recurrent or residual functional tricuspid regurgitation after tricuspid annuloplasty. Circulation 2006;114(1 Suppl):I582–7.

65. Fukuda S, Song JM, Gillinov AM, et al. Tricuspid valve tethering predicts residual tricuspid regurgitation after tricuspid annuloplasty. Circulation 2005; 111(8):975–9.

66. Min SY, Song JM, Kim JH, et al. Geometric changes after tricuspid annuloplasty and predictors of residual tricuspid regurgitation: a real-time three-dimensional echocardiography study. Eur Heart J 2010; 31(23):2871–80.

67. Kalangos A, Sierra J, Beghetti M, et al. Tricuspid valve replacement with a mitral homograft in children with rheumatic tricuspid valvulopathy. J Thorac Cardiovasc Surg 2004;127(6):1682–7.

68. McCarthy PM, Bhudia SK, Rajeswaran J, et al. Tricuspid valve repair: durability and risk factors for failure. J Thorac Cardiovasc Surg 2004;127(3): 674–85.

69. Abdelbar A, Kenawy A, Zacharias J. Minimally invasive tricuspid valve surgery. J Thorac Dis 2021; 13(3):1982–92.

70. Hammerstingl C, Schueler R, Malasa M, et al. Transcatheter treatment of severe tricuspid regurgitation with the MitraClip system. Eur Heart J. Mar 7 2016; 37(10):849–53.

71. Nickenig G, Kowalski M, Hausleiter J, et al. Transcatheter Treatment of Severe Tricuspid Regurgitation With the Edge-to-Edge MitraClip Technique. Circulation 2017;135(19):1802–14.

72. Ruf TF, Hahn RT, Kreidel F, et al. Short-Term Clinical Outcomes of Transcatheter Tricuspid Valve Repair With the Third-Generation MitraClip XTR System. JACC Cardiovasc Interv 2021;14(11): 1231–40.

73. Praz F, Spargias K, Chrissoheris M, et al. Compassionate use of the PASCAL transcatheter mitral valve repair system for patients with severe mitral regurgitation: a multicentre, prospective, observational, first-in-man study. Lancet 2017;390(10096):773–80.

74. Lurz P, Stephan von Bardeleben R, Weber M, et al. Transcatheter Edge-to-Edge Repair for Treatment of Tricuspid Regurgitation. J Am Coll Cardiol 26 2021;77(3):229–39.

75. Kodali S, Hahn RT, Eleid MF, et al. Feasibility Study of the Transcatheter Valve Repair System for Severe Tricuspid Regurgitation. J Am Coll Cardiol 2021; 77(4):345–56.

76. Besler C, Orban M, Rommel KP, et al. Predictors of Procedural and Clinical Outcomes in Patients With Symptomatic Tricuspid Regurgitation Undergoing Transcatheter Edge-to-Edge Repair. JACC Cardiovasc Interv 2018;11(12):1119–28.

77. Liu X, Pu Z, Lim DS, et al. Transcatheter mitral valve repair in a high-surgical risk patient with severe degenerative mitral regurgitation using the novel DragonFly Transcatheter Repair device-First in man implantation in China. Cathet Cardiovasc Interv : official journal of the Society for Cardiac Angiography & Interventions 2021. https://doi.org/10.1002/ccd. 29687.

78. Planer D, Beeri R, Danenberg HD. First-in-Human Transcatheter Tricuspid Valve Repair: 30-Day Follow-Up Experience With the Mistral Device. JACC Cardiovasc Interv 2020;13(18):2091–6.

79. Nickenig G, Weber M, Schuler R, et al. Tricuspid valve repair with the Cardioband system: two-year outcomes of the multicentre, prospective TRI-REPAIR study. EuroIntervention 2021;16(15): e1264–71.

80. Reddy VY, Abbo AR, Ruiz CE, et al. First-in-Human Percutaneous Circumferential Annuloplasty for Secondary Tricuspid Regurgitation. JACC Case reports 2020;2(14):2176–82.

81. Webb JG, Chuang AM, Meier D, et al. Transcatheter Tricuspid Valve Replacement With the EVOQUE System: 1-Year Outcomes of a Multicenter, First-in-Human Experience. JACC Cardiovasc Interv 2022; 15(5):481–91.

82. Kodali S, Hahn RT, George I, et al. Transfemoral Tricuspid Valve Replacement in Patients With Tricuspid Regurgitation: TRISCEND Study 30-Day Results. JACC Cardiovasc Interv 2022;15(5): 471–80.

83. Modine T. Transcatheter tricuspid valve replacement with the LuX-Valve system 1-year results of a multicenter FIH experience. Presented at TVT 2022;8: 2022.

84. Wild MG, Lubos E, Cruz-Gonzalez I, et al. Early Clinical Experience With the TRICENTO Bicaval Valved Stent for Treatment of Symptomatic Severe Tricuspid Regurgitation: A Multicenter Registry. Circ Cardiovasc Interv. Mar 2022;15(3):e011302.

85. Estevez-Loureiro R, Sanchez-Recalde A, Amat-Santos IJ, et al. 6-Month Outcomes of the TricValve System in Patients With Tricuspid Regurgitation: The TRICUS EURO Study. JACC Cardiovasc Interv 2022;15(13):1366–77.

86. Otto CM, Nishimura RA, Bonow RO, et al. 2020 ACC/AHA Guideline for the Management of Patients With Valvular Heart Disease: A Report of the American College of Cardiology/American Heart Association Joint Committee on Clinical Practice Guidelines. Circulation 2021;143(5):e72–227.

Valvular Regurgitation in Adults with Congenital Heart Disease and Heart Failure
Current Status and Potential Interventions

Amrit Misra, MD[a,b,*], Akshay S. Desai, MD[b], Anne Marie Valente, MD[a,b]

KEYWORDS

- Congenital heart disease • Heart failure • Tetralogy of fallot • Fontan • Systemic right ventricle
- Valvular regurgitation

KEY POINTS

- Adult congenital heart disease patients are at risk of developing significant heart failure related to their underlying physiology.
- Valvular regurgitation may lead to significant morbidity and mortality in patients with congenital heart disease.
- Management of valvular regurgitation in congenital heart disease patients with heart failure should be individualized, accounting for the patient's underlying condition, prior interventions, and comorbidities.

INTRODUCTION

Advances in the management of congenital heart disease (CHD) have led to improved life expectancy and outcomes in this patient population. As adult CHD (ACHD) patients grow older, they are at risk of developing heart failure, which is now the leading cause of death in these patients.[1] The causes of heart failure in the ACHD population are multifactorial, including arrhythmias, surgery-related complications, reduced ventricular ejection fraction (EF), diastolic dysfunction, and valvular regurgitation.[2] Although once considered a largely benign residual lesion, it is increasingly being recognized that the presence of significant valvular regurgitation may have a substantial impact on the morbidity and mortality of ACHD patients.[3] In this review, we will describe the etiologies and management strategies for valvular regurgitation in ACHD patients with heart failure.

This chapter will focus on ACHD conditions at high risk for heart failure including tetralogy of Fallot (TOF), Ebstein anomaly, transposition of the great arteries (TGA) with systemic right ventricle (RV), and patients who have undergone the Fontan procedure.

TETRALOGY OF FALLOT
Background

TOF is one of the most common forms of CHD with an incidence of 3 per 10,000 live births.[4] Patients with TOF are born with a ventricular septal defect (VSD), RV hypertrophy, overriding aorta, and RV outflow tract (RVOT) hypertrophy with varying degrees of pulmonary valve hypoplasia (**Fig. 1**). Older adults living with repaired TOF may have first undergone a palliative aorto-pulmonary shunt before the complete repair and are at increased risk of heart failure; however, in the modern era, primary

[a] Department of Cardiology, Boston Children's Hospital, Harvard Medical School, 300 Longwood, Boston, MA 02115, USA; [b] Department of Cardiology, Brigham and Women's Hospital, Harvard Medical School, Boston, MA, USA
* Corresponding author. Boston Adult Congenital Heart Disease Program, Boston Children's Hospital, 300 Longwood Avenue, Boston, MA 02115.
E-mail address: amrit.misra@cardio.chboston.org

Heart Failure Clin 19 (2023) 345–356
https://doi.org/10.1016/j.hfc.2023.02.004
1551-7136/23/© 2023 Elsevier Inc. All rights reserved.

repair of TOF occurs during infancy. For patients for whom the pulmonary valve is significantly hypoplastic, a transannular patch repair is performed, consisting of closure of the VSD, resection of infundibular hypertrophy, and patch augmentation of the pulmonary valve and RVOT.[5] For patients with a competent pulmonary valve, infundibular resection can be done with preservation of the pulmonary valve integrity. However, a vast majority of adults with repaired TOF live with some degree of pulmonary regurgitation (PR).

Etiology of Heart Failure and Valvular Dysfunction

Heart failure affects a significant proportion of patients with repaired TOF, with almost a third of patients reporting dyspnea during adulthood.[6] Heart failure and sudden cardiac death are among the leading causes of mortality in the adult repaired-TOF population.[6] The etiologies of heart failure in the adult patient with repaired TOF are multifactorial and include RV and left ventricular (LV) systolic and/or diastolic dysfunction, tachyarrhythmias, and valvular pathology including significant pulmonary and tricuspid valve regurgitation.[7] PR is common, especially in patients with the transannular patch repair, as the integrity of the native pulmonary valve was disrupted at the time of surgery. Significant PR leads to progressive RV dilation, which in turn can lead to worsening ventricular function due to increased myocardial wall stress (**Fig. 2**).[7] Additionally, dilation of the RV can distort septal geometry, altering ventricular interdependence and resulting in a decline in LV function.[7] It is estimated

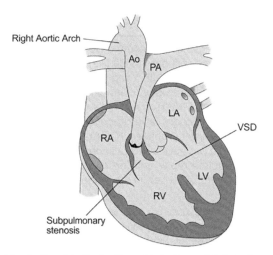

Fig. 1. Graphic illustration of tetralogy of Fallot. Ao, aorta; LA, left atrium; PA, pulmonary artery; RA, right atrium. (Reproduced with permission from OPENPediatrics, Geggel's Congenital Heart Disease Library, edited by Robert Geggel, MD, Boston Children's Hospital.)

that up to 20% of adults with repaired TOF have some degree of LV dysfunction.[8] Right and LV dysfunction have been independently associated with ventricular tachycardia and sudden death in adults with repaired TOF.[9,10]

Adults with repaired TOF may also have varying degrees of tricuspid regurgitation (TR). This may be the result of tricuspid annular dilation, distortion of the valve at the time of TOF repair, injury during device lead placement, or distortion due to infective endocarditis. Severe TR is known to be associated with arrhythmia, death, and heart failure in patients with TOF and leads to worse postprocedural outcomes in those undergoing pulmonary valve replacement.[11,12] Consequently, intervention on the tricuspid valve before regurgitation becomes severe is considered important in reducing morbidity in TOF patients.

Management of Valvular Dysfunction

Timing of pulmonary valve replacement (PVR) in repaired-TOF patients is an area of continued research in ACHD patients. In current guidelines, the severity of PR is determined from cardiac magnetic resonance imaging, with a regurgitation fraction greater than 25% being defined as significant in the American College of Cardiology (ACC) and American Heart Association (AHA) and Canadian guidelines and 30% to 40% in the European guidelines for ACHD management.[13–15] These guidelines advocate for PVR in symptomatic adults with repaired TOF and at least moderate PR. There are also class II recommendations for asymptomatic patients, which involve a combination of indications relating to ventricular dysfunction, RV dilation, or reduced exercise tolerance (**Table 1**).[13–15]

PVR has been associated with symptom improvement, including a change in New York Heart Association class, and reduction in RV volume. However, it has not been shown to reduce mortality or reduce risk of ventricular tachycardia.[16,17] The RV EF does not improve following PVR and can progressively decrease slightly up to 10 years after the intervention.[17,18] These study results highlight the importance of close monitoring and early intervention for patients with significant PR before the development of significant RV dysfunction given patients who already have ventricular dysfunction are unlikely to have improvement in their EF following PVR.

The traditional method for PVR has been surgical intervention, which is associated with an operative mortality of less than 1%. Advances in transcatheter technology over the past 2 decades have resulted in several percutaneous PVR options for

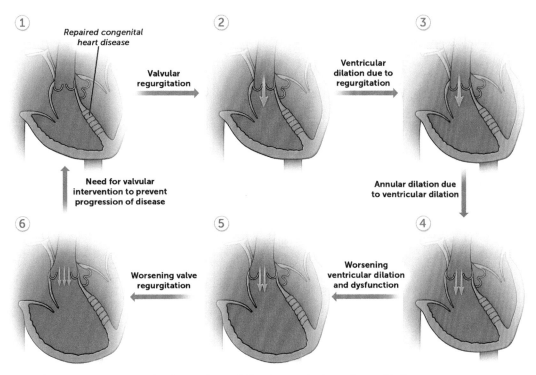

Fig. 2. Pulmonary regurgitation leading to heart failure in repaired tetralogy of Fallot.

both patients with RV to pulmonary artery conduits as well as native outflow tracts.[19,20] The decision whether to pursue surgical or transcatheter valve replacement is individualized based on each patient's anatomy and preference, as adults with significantly dilated RVOT and coronary arteries in close proximity to the RVOT are often not suitable candidates for percutaneous valves.[19]

For TOF patients with severe TR, the indications for intervention are less well defined, with some advocating for intervention for patients with moderate or greater TR and RV dysfunction. Tricuspid valve repair during surgical PVR has been shown to be safe and can lead to improvement in symptoms.[21,22] Transcatheter tricuspid valve replacement (TVR) has been successfully performed in TOF patients with severe TR; however, long-term outcomes for these patients are currently unknown.[23]

EBSTEIN ANOMALY
Background

Ebstein anomaly is present in approximately 1 in 200,000 live births and is caused by a failure of delamination of tricuspid valve leaflets from ventricular myocardium.[24] Subsequently, the tricuspid valve annulus is typically apically displaced, leading to the presence of an "atrialized" RV consisting of ventricular myocardium that is superior to the

tricuspid valve annulus (**Fig. 3**).[24] The anterior leaflet has been classically described as "sail-like" as it compensates for a tethered septal and/or posterior leaflet. Severe TR may develop due to poor coaptation as well as limited mobility of the leaflets. Although classically considered a tricuspid valve condition, it is more appropriate to consider Ebstein anomaly as a RV myopathy. The presentation of patients with Ebstein anomaly is variable and highly dependent on the severity of the valvar pathology; those with mild displacement of the tricuspid valve may have minimal symptoms and present later in life while those with significant valvular pathology may present as infants with heart failure.[25]

Etiology of Heart Failure and Valvular Dysfunction

The lack of coaptation leading to TR can lead to progressive RV dilation with progressive decrease in the RV function, which in turn leads to annular dilation, which leads to worsening TR.[26] It has been reported that up to 64% of adult patients with Ebstein anomaly have moderate or severe tricuspid insufficiency.[27]

The atrialized RV is thin-walled and compliant with limited contractility; hence, patients with large volumes of the atrialized and minimal functional RV are at risk of developing right-sided heart

Table 1
Indications for valve intervention by congenital heart disease type and society guideline

Congenital Heart Disease	American College of Cardiology 2018[13]	Canadian Cardiovascular Society 2022[14]	European Society of Cardiology 2020[15]

Tetralogy of Fallot—pulmonary valve intervention	• Symptomatic patient with ≥moderate PR (RF >25% by CMR) (class I)
	• Asymptomatic patient with ≥moderate PR with two of the following (class IIa):
	  ○ Objective decrease in exercise capacity
	  ○ RV or LV dysfunction
	  ○ RV dilation
	  ○ RVOTO with RVSP > 2/3 systemic pressure
	• Asymptomatic patient with ≥moderate PR and sustained tachyarrhythmias (class IIb)
	• Asymptomatic patient with ≥moderate PR and other lesions requiring surgical interventions (class IIb)
		• Symptomatic patient with severe PR (RF >25% by CMR) (strong)
		• Patients with severe PR and sustained ventricular tachyarrhythmias
		• Asymptomatic patient with severe PR and RV dilation with or without one of the following:
		  ○ RV dysfunction
		  ○ RVOTO
		  ○ Objective decrease in exercise capacity
		• Patients with severe PR who require intervention for other lesions of hemodynamic significance
			• Symptomatic patient with severe PR (RF >30% by CMR) or moderate RVOTO (peak velocity >3 m/s) (class I)
			• Asymptomatic patient with severe PR with one of the following (class IIa):
			  ○ Objective decrease in exercise capacity
			  ○ Progressive RV dilation or moderate TR
			  ○ Progressive RV dysfunction
			  ○ RVOTO with RVSP > 80 mm Hg

Ebstein anomaly—tricuspid valve intervention	• Patient with significant TR with one of the following (class I):
	  ○ Heart failure symptoms
	  ○ Objective decrease in exercise capacity
	• Patient with significant TR with one of the following (class IIa):
	  ○ Systemic desaturation from right-to-left atrial shunt
	  ○ Paradoxic embolism
	  ○ Progressive RV dysfunction
	    Atrial tachyarrhythmias
		• Symptomatic patient with severe TR (strong)
		• Asymptomatic patient with severe TR and one or more of the following:
		  ○ Progressive RV dysfunction or dilation
		  ○ Objective evidence of decreased exercise capacity
		  ○ Oxygen saturation <90% due to R-to-L shunt
		  ○ Paradoxic embolism
		  ○ Refractory atrial arrhythmias
			• Patient with severe TR and symptoms or objective decline in exercise capacity (class I)
			• Asymptomatic patient with progressive RV dilation or reduced RV EF (class IIa)

Transposition of the great arteries—tricuspid valve intervention	D-loop TGA, atrial switch: • N/A Congenitally corrected TGA: • Symptomatic patient with severe TR with preserved or mildly reduced RV EF (class I) • Asymptomatic patient with systemic RV dilation or mildly reduced RV EF (class IIa)	D-loop TGA, atrial switch: • Symptomatic patients with severe TR and RV EF ≥ 45% (strong) Congenitally corrected TGA: • Symptomatic patient with severe TR with preserved or mildly reduced RV EF ≥ 40% (strong) • Asymptomatic patient with systemic RV dilation or mildly reduced RV EF ≥ 40%	D-loop TGA, atrial switch: • Severe TR without significant ventricular systolic dysfunction (EF >40%) regardless of symptoms (class IIa) Congenitally corrected TGA: • Symptomatic patient with severe TR and preserved or mildly impaired systemic RV systolic function (EF > 40%) (class I) • Asymptomatic patient with progressive systemic RV dilation or mildly reduced RV EF >40% (class IIa) • In symptomatic patients with severe TR and more than mildly reduced systemic RV systolic function (EF ≤ 40%) (class IIb)
Fontan procedure—atrioventricular valve intervention	N/A	• Impaired flow dynamics in Fontan circulation/Fontan circulatory dysfunction with ≥ moderate atrioventricular valve regurgitation in the absence of significant ventricular dysfunction	N/A

RV dilation defined as RV end-diastolic volume indexed greater than 160 mL/m^2 or RV end-systolic volume indexed greater than 80 mL/m^2.

Abbreviations: CMR, cardiac magnetic resonance; EF, ejection fraction; LV, left ventricle; N/A, not applicable; PR, pulmonary regurgitation; RF, regurgitant fraction; RV, right ventricle; RVOTO, right ventricular outflow tract obstruction; RVSP, right ventricular systolic pressure; TR, tricuspid regurgitation; TGA, transposition of the great arteries.

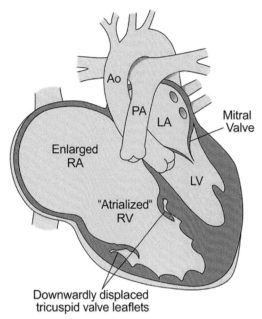

Fig. 3. Graphic illustration of Ebstein anomaly. Ao, aorta; LA, left atrium; PA, pulmonary artery; RA, right atrium. (Reproduced with permission from OPENPediatrics, Geggel's Congenital Heart Disease Library, edited by Robert Geggel, MD, Boston Children's Hospital.)

failure.[13,25] In severe cases, the RV dilation can be significant, leading to distortion of the septal geometry, causing LV dysfunction due to compression of the ventricle from the massively dilated RV.[26] Independent of the RV size, patients with Ebstein anomaly are at risk of developing LV dysfunction, as LV noncompaction has been reported in approximately 20% of cases.[24] Adults with depressed ventricular systolic function, defined as an RV EF less than 41% and LV EF less than 51%, have been associated with higher incidence of sustained ventricular tachycardia, mortality, and transplantation.

Management of Valvular Dysfunction

Indications for tricuspid valve surgery include the presence of moderate or severe TR with symptomatic heart failure, progressive RV dysfunction or dilation, paradoxic embolism, and/or significant recurrent atrial arrhythmias.[13] Previous interventions consisted of manipulation of the valve leaflets to create a monocuspid valve.[28] In the modern era, the Da Silva "cone" repair is increasingly used, often with addition of a tricuspid valve annuloplasty ring in adults.[28] The repair consists of delamination of leaflets from the myocardium, right atrial plication, and the creation of a bicuspid valve by suturing the anterior and posterior leaflets together, with the now-untethered septal valve leaflet completing the valvular apparatus.[28] In

cases of deficient valve leaflet or severe annular dilation, which makes the cone procedure difficult to perform, TVR can be considered.[25,26]

The overall survival after the cone procedure is excellent, with a 93% survival and 99% freedom from operation rate up to 8 years after the procedure.[29] In terms of long-term outcomes, Brown and colleagues reviewed 539 patients from their institution, with TVR performed in ~2 out of 3.[30] While the 30-day mortality was 3%, the 20-year survival was 71.2%.[30] Risk factors for mortality included the presence of moderate-to-severe RV dysfunction, highlighting the importance of intervention before the development of RV failure.[30] Patients who undergo surgery before becoming significantly symptomatic are less likely to have significant cardiac events than their peers who undergo intervention when they are critically ill.[31]

TRANSPOSITION OF THE GREAT ARTERIES WITH SYSTEMIC RIGHT VENTRICLE
Background

Systemic RV (SRV) physiology is characterized by ventriculoarterial discordance, in which the aorta is connected to the RV and the pulmonary artery is attached to the LV.[32] This physiology can be seen in patients with D-loop TGA who have undergone an atrial switch procedure (D-TGA/AS, **Fig. 4**A) or those with physiologically or "congenitally" corrected TGA (cc-TGA) (**Fig. 4**B). The atrial switch procedure is characterized by the creation of intra-atrial baffles that direct systemic venous, deoxygenated blood to a subpulmonary LV and pulmonary venous, oxygenated blood to the SRV.[32] With the advent of improved surgical techniques, the atrial switch was largely replaced by the arterial switch procedure in the 1980s, which connects the discordant arteries to the appropriate ventricles.[32] Patients who have undergone the arterial switch procedure subsequently have anatomically correct ventriculoarterial connections and subpulmonary RVs.

Etiology of Heart Failure and Valvular Dysfunction

The prevalence of ventricular dysfunction is common in the SRV population; up to 50% of patients with cc-TGA can develop SRV dysfunction by the age of 40 years.[33] The chronic systemic afterload on a compliant RV designed to pump to the low-pressure pulmonary circulation leads to progressive ventricular dilation and hypertrophy, which in turn can contribute to myocardial fibrosis and ischemia, leading to RV dysfunction.[34] Goal-directed medical therapy traditionally used for patients with structurally normal hearts and cardiomyopathy including

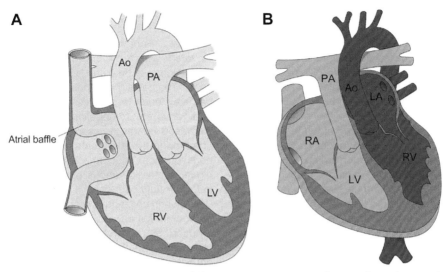

Fig. 4. Graphic illustration of (*A*) transposition of the great arteries, status after atrial switch procedure, and (*B*) congenitally corrected transposition of the great arteries. Ao, aorta; LA, left atrium; PA, pulmonary artery; RA, right atrium. (Reproduced with permission from OPENPediatrics, Geggel's Congenital Heart Disease Library, edited by Robert Geggel, MD, Boston Children's Hospital.)

beta-blockers and angiotensinogen-converting enzyme inhibitors are commonly used for these patients; however, there is no conclusive evidence that these agents affect long-term outcomes in SRV patients.[35] This may be related to a small sample size and surrogate endpoints that have been chosen in these studies.

Tricuspid valve regurgitation is the most common valvular pathology seen in SRV patients, with at least moderate TR in 25% of patients.[36] The primary mechanism is annular dilation secondary to ventricular dilation, leading to limited coaptation of the valve leaflets.[32] Tricuspid valve dysplasia is common in cc-TGA patients and contributes to TR.[32] The presence of TR can lead to additional volume load and strain on a dysfunctional SRV, leading to further RV dilation, resulting in increased annular dilation and worsening TR. This viscous cycle can increase the morbidity and mortality of SRV patients; as severe TR has been shown to be independently associated with heart failure hospitalizations, mortality, and decreased transplant-free survival in the D-TGA/AS population.[36–38]

Management of Valvular Dysfunction

Recognizing the risk of decompensation with severe regurgitation, prompt assessment, and intervention for these patients is essential to prevent long-term complications. TVR for symptomatic patients with severe TR, cc-TGA, and preserved SRV function is a class I recommendation in the 2018 ACC/AHA guidelines; class IIa recommendations include TVR for patients with severe TR with SRV dilation or dysfunction.[13] The European Society of Cardiology ACHD guidelines recommend consideration of TVR or repair for asymptomatic patients with an SRV ejection EF greater than 40%.[15] The 2022 Canadian guidelines for ACHD management have a strong recommendation for symptomatic patients with cc-TGA with severe TR and preserved or mildly reduced RV EF ≥ 40%.[14]

The frequency of tricuspid valve repair in patients with TGA who have undergone the atrial switch procedure is lower. In one study of 454 patients, with a maximal mean age at follow-up of 31.5 years, 10 patients (2.2%) required TVR or repair.[37]

Overall outcomes after TVR for the SRV population are acceptable if surgery occurs before significant ventricular dysfunction develops. Mongeon and colleagues showed that SRV EF less than 40% at the time of tricuspid valve surgery associated with an increase in late mortality, highlighting the importance of early tricuspid valve intervention.[39] Tricuspid valve surgery can lead to improvement in symptoms and prevent worsening RV function.[40]

FONTAN PROCEDURE
Background

Patients with complex forms of CHD may have anatomy and physiology requiring them to undergo a series of surgeries culminating in the Fontan procedure. Common diagnoses include tricuspid atresia and hypoplastic left heart syndrome

(HLHS). The first stage of surgical palliation may involve a systemic artery to pulmonary artery shunt (modified Blalock Taussig or Sano shunt), followed by a procedure called the bidirectional Glenn, in which the superior vena cava (SVC) is connected to the pulmonary arteries. Completion of the Fontan requires that both the SVC and inferior vena cava are anastomosed directed to the pulmonary arteries to deliver deoxygenated blood to the lungs, with the pulmonary veins draining oxygenated blood to essentially a common atrium. Oxygenated blood drains through the systemic atrioventricular valve to the single ventricle, which connects to the systemic circulation (**Fig. 5**A).[41] Typically, the bidirectional Glenn procedure occurs around 4 months of age with Fontan completion by 2 to 3 years of age. For patients with HLHS, an additional procedure, known as the Norwood procedure, is performed during the first week of life to connect the functioning RV to the aorta (**Fig. 5**B).

The Fontan procedure has led to significant improvement in survival for single-ventricle patients. Before the advent of the procedure, the survival at 10 years of life was approximately 10%; following the widespread implementation of these surgical techniques, the 10- and 20-year survival have been estimated to be as high as 90% and 74%, respectively.[42,43]

Etiology of Heart Failure and Valvular Dysfunction

Multiple complications can develop secondary to the underlying physiology, including the development of "Fontan failure." Patients with a failing Fontan can exhibit symptoms of right-sided heart failure, including lower-extremity edema and ascites, as well as extra-cardiac manifestations including protein-losing enteropathy and plastic bronchitis.[42] The etiology of Fontan failure is multifactorial; Fontan pressures are chronically elevated, with a mean pressure of 12 to 15 mm Hg, which over time can lead to diastolic dysfunction.[44] The passive, nonpulsatile flow of the Fontan pathway leads to progressive venous congestion and adverse remodeling, further leading to increased Fontan pressures.[44] Hepatic fibrosis is common in these patients and is thought to be a consequence of congestive hepatopathy from higher systemic venous pressures, which results in further fluid overload.[44]

Book and colleagues proposed four phenotypes of Fontan failure, which included patients with reduced or preserved EF, normal function and pressures, and abnormal lymphatic drainage.[42] In patients referred for heart transplantation, ventricular dysfunction is common and can be seen in up to 60% of patients.[41,45] Patients with both preserved and reduced EF are traditionally treated with standard goal-directed medical therapy used for LV systolic and diastolic dysfunction, including diuretics, aldosterone antagonists, beta-blockers, and angiotensin-converting enzyme inhibitors. The other two phenotypes of Fontan failure have been traditionally difficult to manage given the limited utility of heart failure medications for these phenotypes. Therapeutics including lymphatic interventions and pulmonary vasodilators have been attempted to ameliorate the symptoms associated with these subsets of heart failure.[42]

Atrioventricular valve regurgitation (AVVR) is common in Fontan patients, with up to 20% having at least moderate regurgitation during childhood.[46] Up to 60% of patients may develop significant AV valve regurgitation by 25 years.[47] There are multiple

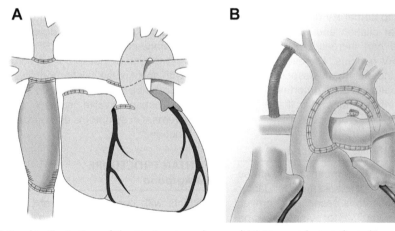

Fig. 5. (*A*) Graphic illustration of the Fontan procedure and (*B*) Norwood procedure. (Reproduced with permission from OPENPediatrics, Geggel's Congenital Heart Disease Library, edited by Robert Geggel, MD, Boston Children's Hospital.)

etiologies for the development of AVVR, which include annular dilation secondary to ventricular dysfunction and anatomic abnormalities of the valve, including leaflet tethering or prolapse.[48,49]

The presence of moderate or worse AVVR is a risk factor for the development of Fontan failure. King and colleagues demonstrated that patients with significant AVVR were twice as likely to have Fontan failure compared to their counterparts without AVVR.[47] Forty-six percent of patients with AVVR had Fontan failure at 20 years of follow-up compared to 23% of patients without significant AVVR.[47] Patients with RV morphology of their single ventricle, such as those with HLHS, and more than moderate AVVR have a 2.8 times higher chance of death or requiring transplantation than their peers with mild AVVR.[50]

Management of Valvular Dysfunction

There is a paucity of guidelines for intervention for atrioventricular valve dysfunction in Fontan patients. The Canadian guidelines do suggest intervention in those patients with impaired flow dynamics in the Fontan circulation with at lease moderate AVVR in the absence of significant ventricular dysfunction.[14] This recommendation mirrors that for other forms of CHD, where it has been recognized that it is optimal to intervene on severe AVVR before the development of ventricular dysfunction.[48] Interventions for the failing atrioventricular valve include annuloplasty, commissurotomy, or valve replacement.[48]

Despite advances in surgical technique, the success rate for patients who require atrioventricular valve intervention can be poor for patients with significant comorbidities. The mortality following surgical intervention for AVVR is high, with 1- and 10-year survival of 72% and 61% in the pediatric population, respectively[51]; another study found the 15-year postsurgery survival to be 45%.[52] King and colleagues reported that the rates of atrioventricular valve repair failure, defined as a reoperation or development of at least moderate AVVR, were 32%, 37%, and 50% at 5, 10, and 20 years, respectively, after the first surgical intervention.[47]

SUMMARY

ACHD patients can develop significant heart failure, which is worsened by the valvular regurgitation. Significant valvular regurgitation has been shown to be associated with worse outcomes in ACHD patients. Current guidelines, summarized in **Table 1**, largely recommend valvular interventions in symptomatic ACHD patients; however, recognizing the lack of improvement of ventricular performance following valve intervention, both transcatheter and

surgical options should be considered earlier in these complex patients particularly while ventricular function is preserved.

CLINICS CARE POINTS

- Pulmonary regurgitation is common in patients with repaired TOF and can lead to right-sided heart failure due to worsening right ventricular volume overload and dysfunction.

- Tricuspid valve regurgitation can exacerbate right ventricular dysfunction in TOF patients and is associated with worse outcomes.

- Indications for PVR for TOF patients include symptoms or progressive right ventricular dilation or dysfunction.

- PVR leads to improvement in symptoms and a reduction in right ventricular volume; it has not been shown to reduce mortality or the incidence of ventricular arrhythmias.

- Indications for tricuspid valve intervention in TOF patients are not well defined; tricuspid valve repair during PVR has been associated with improved outcomes for select patients.

- Patients with Ebstein anomaly are at risk of developing heart failure secondary to right ventricular dysfunction and dilation due to secondary tricuspid valve regurgitation and poor ventricular contractility.

- Left ventricular dysfunction may be present in patients with Ebstein anomaly due to left ventricular noncompaction or distortion in the septal geometry from right ventricular volume overload.

- Indications for surgical intervention on the tricuspid valve in Ebstein anomaly are progressive RV dysfunction/dilation, heart failure, and recurrent atrial arrhythmias.

- Surgical outcomes for tricuspid valve surgery for Ebstein anomaly are excellent if the interventions occur before patients develop significant right or left ventricular dysfunction.

- Patients with SRV are at high risk of developing ventricular dysfunction and TR.

- Severe TR in SRV patients is an independent risk factor for heart failure hospitalization, mortality, and decreased time to transplantation.

- Current guidelines recommend tricuspid valve replacement or repair for patients with symptomatic tricuspid regurgitation; consideration of tricuspid valve repair or replacement is recommended for asymptomatic patients with severe tricuspid regurgitation and SRV dilation or dysfunction.

- Outcomes after tricuspid replacement in the SRV population are generally favorable for patients with preserved right ventricular function.
- Patients with single ventricle physiology are at high risk of developing Fontan failure, which includes patients with both reduced and preserved systolic function.
- AVVR is common among Fontan patients and is a risk factor for Fontan failure.
- There are no current guidelines regarding the optimal time to intervene on a failing atrioventricular valve for Fontan patients; atrioventricular valve intervention should be considered for patients with severe regurgitation with preserved or worsening ventricular function.

DISCLOSURE

The authors have nothing to disclose.

ACKNOWLEDGEMENT

A.M. Valente is on the advisory board for Practice Update (Elsevier) and is supported by the Sarah M. Liamos Fund for Adult Congenital Heart Disease Research.

REFERENCES

1. Nieminen HP, Jokinen EV, Sairanen HI. Causes of late deaths after pediatric cardiac surgery: a population-based study. J Am Coll Cardiol 2007; 50(13):1263–71.
2. Sabanayagam A, Cavus O, Williams J, et al. Management of Heart Failure in Adult Congenital Heart Disease. Heart Fail Clin 2018;14(4):569–77.
3. Alsaied T, Bokma JP, Engel ME, et al. Predicting long-term mortality after Fontan procedures: A risk score based on 6707 patients from 28 studies. Congenit Heart Dis 2017;12(4):393–8.
4. Bailliard F, Anderson RH. Tetralogy of Fallot. Orphanet J Rare Dis 2009;4:2.
5. Krieger EV, Valente AM. Tetralogy of Fallot. Cardiol Clin 2020;38(3):365–77.
6. Nollert G, Fischlein T, Bouterwek S, et al. Long-term survival in patients with repair of tetralogy of Fallot: 36-year follow-up of 490 survivors of the first year after surgical repair. J Am Coll Cardiol 1997;30(5): 1374–83.
7. Wald RM, Valente AM, Marelli A. Heart failure in adult congenital heart disease: Emerging concepts with a focus on tetralogy of Fallot. Trends Cardiovasc Med 2015;25(5):422–32.
8. Broberg CS, Aboulhosn J, Mongeon FP, et al. Prevalence of left ventricular systolic dysfunction in adults with repaired tetralogy of fallot. Am J Cardiol 2011;107(8):1215–20.
9. Valente AM, Gauvreau K, Assenza GE, et al. Contemporary predictors of death and sustained ventricular tachycardia in patients with repaired tetralogy of Fallot enrolled in the INDICATOR cohort. Heart 2014;100(3):247–53.
10. Ghai A, Silversides C, Harris L, et al. Left ventricular dysfunction is a risk factor for sudden cardiac death in adults late after repair of tetralogy of Fallot. J Am Coll Cardiol 2002;40(9):1675–80.
11. Bokma JP, Winter MM, Oosterhof T, et al. Severe tricuspid regurgitation is predictive for adverse events in tetralogy of Fallot. Heart 2015;101(10): 794–9 (In eng).
12. Woudstra OI, Bokma JP, Winter MM, et al. Clinical course of tricuspid regurgitation in repaired tetralogy of Fallot. Int J Cardiol 2017;243:191–3.
13. Stout KK, Daniels CJ, Aboulhosn JA, et al. 2018 AHA/ACC Guideline for the Management of Adults With Congenital Heart Disease: Executive Summary: A Report of the American College of Cardiology/ American Heart Association Task Force on Clinical Practice Guidelines. Circulation 2019;139(14): e637–97.
14. Marelli A, Beauchesne L, Colman J, et al. Canadian Cardiovascular Society 2022 Guidelines for Cardiovascular Interventions in Adults With Congenital Heart Disease. Can J Cardiol 2022;38(7):862–96.
15. Baumgartner H, De Backer J. The ESC Clinical Practice Guidelines for the Management of Adult Congenital Heart Disease 2020. Eur Heart J 2020; 41(43):4153–4.
16. Harrild DM, Berul CI, Cecchin F, et al. Pulmonary valve replacement in tetralogy of Fallot: impact on survival and ventricular tachycardia. Circulation 2009;119(3):445–51.
17. Mongeon FP, Ben Ali W, Khairy P, et al. Pulmonary Valve Replacement for Pulmonary Regurgitation in Adults With Tetralogy of Fallot: A Meta-analysis-A Report for the Writing Committee of the 2019 Update of the Canadian Cardiovascular Society Guidelines for the Management of Adults With Congenital Heart Disease. Can J Cardiol 2019;35(12):1772–83.
18. Hallbergson A, Gauvreau K, Powell AJ, et al. Right ventricular remodeling after pulmonary valve replacement: early gains, late losses. Ann Thorac Surg 2015;99(2):660–6.
19. Alkashkari W, Alsubei A, Hijazi ZM. Transcatheter Pulmonary Valve Replacement: Current State of Art. Curr Cardiol Rep 2018;20(4):27.
20. McElhinney DB, Zhang Y, Levi DS, et al. Reintervention and Survival After Transcatheter Pulmonary Valve Replacement. J Am Coll Cardiol 2022;79(1): 18–32.
21. Roubertie F, Seguela PE, Jalal Z, et al. Tricuspid valve repair and pulmonary valve replacement in

adults with repaired tetralogy of Fallot. J Thorac Cardiovasc Surg 2017;154(1):214–23.

22. Deshaies C, Trottier H, Khairy P, et al. Tricuspid Intervention Following Pulmonary Valve Replacement in Adults With Congenital Heart Disease. J Am Coll Cardiol 2020;75(9):1033–43.
23. Challa A, Markham R, Walters D. Percutaneous valve in valve in the tricuspid position in a patient with Tetralogy of Fallot. BMJ Case Rep 2017;2017.
24. Attenhofer Jost CH, Connolly HM, Dearani JA, et al. Ebstein's anomaly. Circulation 2007;115(2):277–85.
25. Dearani JA, Mora BN, Nelson TJ, et al. Ebstein anomaly review: what's now, what's next? Expert Rev Cardiovasc Ther 2015;13(10):1101–9.
26. Schultz K, Haeffele CL. Heart failure in the adult Ebstein patient. Heart Fail Rev 2020;25(4):623–32.
27. Attie F, Rosas M, Rijlaarsdam M, et al. The adult patient with Ebstein anomaly. Outcome in 72 unoperated patients. Medicine (Baltim) 2000;79(1):27–36.
28. Perier P, Pajak J, Pawlak S, et al. Ebstein's anomaly-How to correct severe anatomical forms of the defect in adults. Ann Cardiothorac Surg 2017;6(3):287–9.
29. Holst KA, Dearani JA, Said S, et al. Improving Results of Surgery for Ebstein Anomaly: Where Are We After 235 Cone Repairs? Ann Thorac Surg 2018;105(1):160–8.
30. Brown ML, Dearani JA, Danielson GK, et al. The outcomes of operations for 539 patients with Ebstein anomaly. J Thorac Cardiovasc Surg 2008;135(5):1120–36, 1136 e1-e1136.
31. Homzova L, Photiadis J, Sinzobahamvya N, et al. Surgical management of Ebstein anomaly: impact of the adult congenital heart disease anatomical and physiological classifications. Interact Cardiovasc Thorac Surg 2021;32(4):593–600.
32. Brida M, Diller GP, Gatzoulis MA. Systemic Right Ventricle in Adults With Congenital Heart Disease: Anatomic and Phenotypic Spectrum and Current Approach to Management. Circulation 2018;137(5):508–18.
33. Graham TP Jr, Bernard YD, Mellen BG, et al. Long-term outcome in congenitally corrected transposition of the great arteries: a multi-institutional study. J Am Coll Cardiol 2000;36(1):255–61.
34. Andrade L, Carazo M, Wu F, et al. Mechanisms for heart failure in systemic right ventricle. Heart Fail Rev 2020;25(4):599–607.
35. Zaragoza-Macias E, Zaidi AN, Dendukuri N, et al. Medical Therapy for Systemic Right Ventricles: A Systematic Review (Part 1) for the 2018 AHA/ACC Guideline for the Management of Adults With Congenital Heart Disease: A Report of the American College of Cardiology/American Heart Association Task Force on Clinical Practice Guidelines. Circulation 2019;139(14):e801–13.
36. Broberg CS, van Dissel A, Minnier J, et al. Long-Term Outcomes After Atrial Switch Operation for Transposition of the Great Arteries. J Am Coll Cardiol 2022;80(10):951–63.
37. Antonova P, Rohn V, Chaloupecky V, et al. Predictors of mortality after atrial correction of transposition of the great arteries. Heart 2022. https://doi.org/10.1136/heartjnl-2021-320035.
38. Woudstra OI, Zandstra TE, Vogel RF, et al. Clinical Course Long After Atrial Switch: A Novel Risk Score for Major Clinical Events. J Am Heart Assoc 2021;10(5):e018565.
39. Mongeon FP, Connolly HM, Dearani JA, et al. Congenitally corrected transposition of the great arteries ventricular function at the time of systemic atrioventricular valve replacement predicts long-term ventricular function. J Am Coll Cardiol 2011;57(20):2008–17.
40. Koolbergen DR, Ahmed Y, Bouma BJ, et al. Follow-up after tricuspid valve surgery in adult patients with systemic right ventricles. Eur J Cardio Thorac Surg 2016;50(3):456–63.
41. Rychik J, Atz AM, Celermajer DS, et al. Evaluation and Management of the Child and Adult With Fontan Circulation: A Scientific Statement From the American Heart Association. Circulation 2019. CIR0000000000000696.
42. Book WM, Gerardin J, Saraf A, et al. Clinical Phenotypes of Fontan Failure: Implications for Management. Congenit Heart Dis 2016;11(4):296–308.
43. Downing TE, Allen KY, Glatz AC, et al. Long-term survival after the Fontan operation: Twenty years of experience at a single center. J Thorac Cardiovasc Surg 2017;154(1):243–253 e2.
44. Kumar TKS. The failing Fontan. Indian J Thorac Cardiovasc Surg 2021;37(Suppl 1):82–90.
45. Griffiths ER, Kaza AK, Wyler von Ballmoos MC, et al. Evaluating failing Fontans for heart transplantation: predictors of death. Ann Thorac Surg 2009;88(2):558–63 [discussion: 563-4].
46. Anderson PA, Sleeper LA, Mahony L, et al. Contemporary outcomes after the Fontan procedure: a Pediatric Heart Network multicenter study. J Am Coll Cardiol 2008;52(2):85–98.
47. King G, Ayer J, Celermajer D, et al. Atrioventricular Valve Failure in Fontan Palliation. J Am Coll Cardiol 2019;73(7):810–22.
48. Tseng SY, Siddiqui S, Di Maria MV, et al. Atrioventricular Valve Regurgitation in Single Ventricle Heart Disease: A Common Problem Associated With Progressive Deterioration and Mortality. J Am Heart Assoc 2020;9(11):e015737.
49. Takahashi K, Inage A, Rebeyka IM, et al. Real-time 3-dimensional echocardiography provides new insight into mechanisms of tricuspid valve regurgitation in patients with hypoplastic left heart syndrome. Circulation 2009;120(12):1091–8.

50. King G, Buratto E, Celermajer DS, et al. Natural and Modified History of Atrioventricular Valve Regurgitation in Patients With Fontan Circulation. J Am Coll Cardiol 2022;79(18):1832–45.

51. Wong DJ, Iyengar AJ, Wheaton GR, et al. Long-term outcomes after atrioventricular valve operations in patients undergoing single-ventricle palliation. Ann Thorac Surg 2012;94(2):606–13 [discussion: 613].

52. Menon SC, Dearani JA, Cetta F. Long-term outcome after atrioventricular valve surgery following modified Fontan operation. Cardiol Young 2011;21(1): 83–8.

Arrythmia-Mediated Valvular Heart Disease

Sébastien Deferm, MD, PhD[a,b], Philippe B. Bertrand, MD PhD[a,c], Sebastiaan Dhont, MD[a,c], Ralph S. von Bardeleben, MD[b], Pieter M. Vandervoort, MD[a,c],*

KEYWORDS

- Atrial functional mitral regurgitation • Atrial functional tricuspid regurgitation • Atrial fibrillation
- Atrial myopathy • Functional mitral regurgitation • Heart failure with preserved ejection fraction
- Isolated tricuspid regurgitation • Left atrium

KEY POINTS

- Atrial functional mitral and tricuspid regurgitation (AFMR and AFTR) are two manifestations of atrio-ventricular disease, driven by atrial and annular pathology in the context of atrial fibrillation and heart failure with preserved ejection fraction.
- Annular dilation pulls the leaflets apart which typically results in a central coaptation defect when the increase in leaflet length fails to match annular dilation.
- Echocardiography is key to discern AFMR and AFTR from their ventricular counterparts, given different underlying pathophysiology, prognosis, and treatment needs. However, considerable overlap may appear in the "functional MR-spectrum."
- The question remains if poor outcomes are driven by regurgitation itself or rather the underlying atrial myopathy or a combination of both. Especially in the era of transcatheter therapy, knowing "who" and "when" to treat is vital, after careful etiology adjudication.
- Care should be taken with the term "isolated tricuspid regurgitation" given that this wording can serve multiple connotations.

INTRODUCTION

Atrial fibrillation (AF) is the most common sustained cardiac arrhythmia worldwide, estimated to afflict over 30 million people in 2010.[1] In the United States alone, estimates of the prevalence ranged from 2.7 to 6.1 million in 2010,[2,3] with projections to reach nearly 12.1 million or higher in 2030,[4] justifying the term "global pandemic." This unfavorable trend is largely explained by aging of the population, improved survival as well as an increase in comorbidities and cardiovascular risk factors.[3,5] The accompanying increase in morbidity and mortality with large socioeconomic impact has led to a paradigm shift in diagnosis and management of AF.

Among others, huge efforts have been made in stroke and heart failure prevention for patients with AF, given their close association.[5] Furthermore, it is well-known that virtually every significant valvular lesion can be associated with the development of AF. Arrhythmia-mediated atrioventricular valve disease (ie, AF as the inciting mechanism for atrioventricular valve disease) has received far less attention, in spite of recent data underscoring its importance in daily clinical practice and adverse impact on prognosis.[6-9] This chapter particularly focuses on atrial functional mitral and tricuspid regurgitation (AFMR and AFTR), two manifestations of AF and atrial myopathy.

[a] Hasselt University, Agoralaan Building D, 3590 Diepenbeek, Belgium; [b] Department of Cardiology, Mainz University Hospital, Langenbeckstraße 1, Mainz, Germany; [c] Department of Cardiology, Hospital Oost-Limburg Genk, Schiepse Bos 6, 3600 Genk, Belgium
* Corresponding author. Schiepse bos 6, 3600 Genk, Belgium.
E-mail address: pieter.vandervoort@zol.be
Twitter: @S_Deferm (S.D.); @Ph_Bertrand (P.B.B.); @S_Dhont (S.D.); @vonbardelebenRS (R.S.B.); @pietvandervoort (P.M.V.)

Heart Failure Clin 19 (2023) 357–377
https://doi.org/10.1016/j.hfc.2023.02.008
1551-7136/23/© 2023 Elsevier Inc. All rights reserved.

NATURE OF THE PROBLEM IN ATRIAL FUNCTIONAL MITRAL REGURGITATION

Traditionally, secondary or ventricular functional mitral regurgitation (VFMR) is believed to result from a *functional imbalance* between increased leaflet tethering forces and decreased left ventricular (LV) closing forces in the setting of a structurally normal mitral valve apparatus[10,11] (**Fig. 1**). Typically, this scenario sets stage in the context of adverse LV remodeling and often portends poor prognosis. The ensuing left atrial (LA) volume load can concomitantly induce some mitral annular (MA) enlargement, which on its turn adversely affects leaflet coaptation.[6]

Currently, there is a growing understanding that functional mitral and/or tricuspid regurgitation (TR) may also relate to isolated atrial pathology, even in the absence of ventricular disease. This so-called "atrial functional mitral regurgitation" (AFMR) is typically observed in AF and/or heart failure with preserved ejection fraction (HFpEF)[6,12] (see **Fig. 1**; **Fig. 2**). A key element in its pathophysiology is the concept of "annular-leaflet imbalance," carefully balanced by the degree of annular dilation/dysfunction as well as (mal)-adaptive leaflet growth. Gertz and colleagues[13] were among the first to independently link LA and MA dimensions to functional mitral regurgitation (MR) in a small cohort of elderly patients referred for pulmonary vein isolation. Importantly, only those who successfully maintained sinus rhythm at follow-up showed a significant reduction in MR, attributed to shrinkage of the LA and MA (**Fig. 3**). This led to believe that MA dilation is an integral component

affecting normal leaflet coaptation in the pathophysiology of this Carpentier type I MR (**Fig. 4**).[14] These findings were conflicted by other mechanistic studies,[15,16] claiming annular dilation alone is insufficient to cause clinically meaningful MR.

The controversy is explained by the process of adaptive leaflet growth. Leaflet traction by excessive annular dilation activates the transforming growth factor beta (TGFβ) signaling pathway, which on its turn promotes compensatory leaflet growth. Two recent studies noted that compensatory leaflet growth invariably fails to match extreme annular dilation (annular area >8 cm/m²). However, large heterogeneity in AFMR-severity was found in those with moderately dilated annular area (5–8 cm/m²). Particularly, in this subgroup, the amount of compensatory leaflet growth seemed to be the decisive factor whether or not malcoaptation occurred.[17–19] Hence, not annular dilation per se, but rather annular-leaflet *imbalance* defines AFMR (**Fig. 5**). Along with leaflet growth, overactivation of the TGFβ pathway also induces unwanted leaflet thickening[20] and fibrosis[21] which may restrict leaflet motion (the addition of a so-called "organic contribution").[22] Some reports suggest this molecular pathway will become a future treatment target,[23,24] in view of promoting leaflet growth while avoiding thickening.

In addition, abnormalities in MA structure and function play an important role in the pathogenesis of AFMR. The fibrous constitution of the saddle-shaped MA precludes any intrinsic motion. Instead, sphincter-like annular contraction is governed by the motion of adjacent atrial and ventricular musculature. Subtle impairments in (pre-)

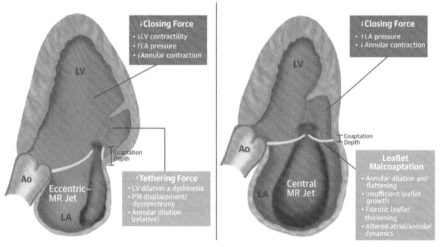

Fig. 1. Ventricular functional (left-sided panel) versus atrial functional MR (right-sided panel). Ao, aorta; LA, left atrium; LV, left ventricle; MR, mitral regurgitation; PM, papillary muscle. (*From* Deferm S, Bertrand PB, Verbrugge FH, et al. Atrial Functional Mitral Regurgitation: JACC Review Topic of the Week. J Am Coll Cardiol. 2019;73(19):2465-2476.)

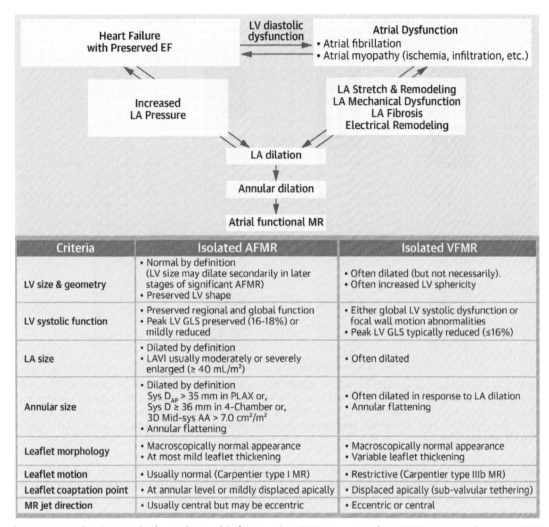

Fig. 2. Key mechanisms and echocardiographic features in AFMR, as opposed to VFMR. AA, annular area; AFMR, atrial functional mitral regurgitation; LA, left atrium; LAVI, left atrial volume index; LV, left ventricle/ventricular; LV GLS, left ventricular global longitudinal strain; MR, mitral regurgitation; VFMR, ventricular functional mitral regurgitation. (*From* Zoghbi WA, Levine RA, Flachskampf F, et al. Atrial Functional Mitral Regurgitation: A JACC: Cardiovascular Imaging Expert Panel Viewpoint. JACC Cardiovasc Imaging. 2022;15(11):1870-1882.)

systolic atrial and annular dynamics during persisting AF negatively influence the ongoing systolic annular-leaflet imbalance as normal leaflet apposition is hampered.[25,26] Sinus rhythm restoration allows for a gradual recovery of these mechanics, followed by a significant reduction in effective regurgitant orifice area (EROA) as coaptation is reinforced independent of LA remodeling[26] (**Fig. 6**).

Finally, some investigators reported on posterior leaflet tethering in subjects with extreme atrial dilation. In giant left atria, the posterior MA is drawn toward the epicardial surface of the posterobasal LV wall. The posterior mitral valve leaflet—attached to this part of the annulus—is pulled along with it, which on its turn increases the annulo-papillary distance and causes "atriogenic leaflet tethering"[7,18,27] (**Fig. 7**). This rare form of AFMR has been mostly described in Asian literature with trends toward worse outcomes.[8]

As highlighted above, HFpEF and/or AF represent two common clinical scenarios leading to excessive LA and MA dilation in the context of preserved left ventricular ejection fraction (LVEF).[6] Both syndromes are closely related with LA myopathy as a common pathogenic driver,[28,29] next to shared cardiovascular risk factors (**Fig. 8**). Chronic LA hypertension in the context of ensuing diastolic dysfunction induces LA spherical deformation, interstitial fibrosis, and functional impairment, even in those who maintain sinus rhythm.[7,30] Furthermore, the presence of atrial

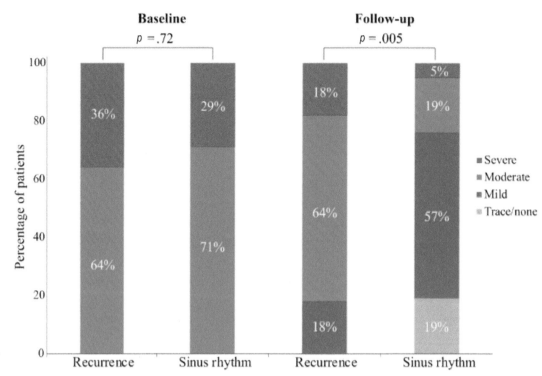

Fig. 3. Subcategorization according to rhythm status following catheter ablation for persistent AF. Eigthy-two percent in the recurrence group (*n* = 11) still showed significant MR compared with 24% in the group who maintained sinus rhythm at follow-up (*n* = 21). (*From* Gertz ZM, Raina A, Saghy L, et al. Evidence of atrial functional mitral regurgitation due to atrial fibrillation: reversal with arrhythmia control. J Am Coll Cardiol. 2011;58(14):1474-1481.)

dysfunction may predispose to new-onset AF, which by itself worsens adverse remodeling ("AF begets AF")[28] and overall outcomes in HFpEF. This is touted by the high prevalence of occult

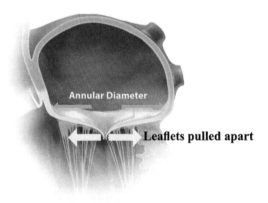

Fig. 4. Excessive annular dilation pulls both mitral valve leaflets apart, which typically inflicts a central regurgitant jet. (This article was published in Struct Heart. 2021, Volume 5 (3), Yap J, Bolling SF, Rogers JH, Contemporary Review in Interventional Cardiology: Mitral Annuloplasty in Secondary Mitral Regurgitation, 247-262, Copyright Elsevier 2021.)

HFpEF among subjects with AF, especially those who remain symptomatic after sinus rhythm restoration.[31] Another example includes the growing literature emphasizing the relevance of a distinct HFpEF phenotype with more advanced LA myopathy disproportionate to the degree of LV dysfunction.[30–33] Importantly, this so-called LA/AF predominant phenotype is particularly prone to develop AFMR, which naturally leaves to question whether morbidity and mortality are driven by AFMR or rather by the underlying myopathy.[34] One study by Tamargo and colleagues[34] noted moderate or worse AFMR to be associated with worse hemodynamics, exercise reserve, and overall outcomes. Nevertheless, this association faded after incorporating LA myopathy (measured by peak atrial longitudinal reservoir strain) into the regression model, which could suggest that the underlying LA myopathy is more important than AFMR itself.[34] Also, one recent study found some patients with AFMR show a blunted hemodynamic response after transcatheter edge-to-edge repair (TEER), even when adequate MR reduction was achieved.[35,36] Possible invasive measurements of LA pressure and v-wave can identify different subgroups. Most likely, a

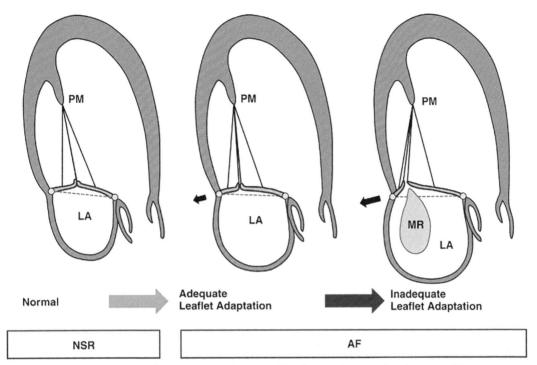

Fig. 5. Schematic presentation of AFMR-progression. Mitral leaflet area increase has the potential to compensate for annular dilation in AF. When leaflet growth fails to match annular dilation, AFMR appears. AFMR, atrial functional mitral regurgitation; LA, left atrium; MR, mitral regurgitation; NSR, normal sinus rhythm; PM, papillary muscle. (*From* Kim DH, Heo R, Handschumacher MD, et al. Mitral Valve Adaptation to Isolated Annular Dilation: Insights Into the Mechanism of Atrial Functional Mitral Regurgitation. *JACC Cardiovasc Imaging*. 2019;12(4):665-677.)

bidirectional relationship between AFMR and LA myopathy exists.[34] Recent cross-sectional data fall short in unraveling the sequence of causality between AFMR, LA myopathy, and HFpEF.[7] The finesses of this intriguing question are further discussed below in the section on "Epidemiology and Clinical Outcomes."

EPIDEMIOLOGY AND CLINICAL OUTCOMES OF ATRIAL FUNCTIONAL MITRAL REGURGITATION

Previously reported prevalence numbers are quite variable, owing to the large granularity of AFMR definitions[7] and the fact that MR represents a "disease spectrum" rather than invariably being constituted of completely distinct subtypes.[35] Therefore, a newly released expert panel viewpoint paper sought to provide a more standardized definition of AFMR.[7]

According to recent epidemiological data, nearly one in three cases of clinically significant moderate-to-severe MR was attributed to AFMR.[9] Women of advanced age, with a broad range of comorbidities, were typically affected. Over 50% showed a history of AF/atrial flutter, underscoring

the close interrelation between atrial rhythm disorders and AFMR, unequaled in any other MR form. Remarkably, although this group shared comparable ranges of LVEF with degenerative MR (DMR), they contrasted with worse diastolic indices and significantly more heart failure events in spite lower regurgitant volumes (mean EROA only 0.20 ± 0.08 cm^2 in AFMR). Similar findings were obtained in one additional retrospective study[8] exclusively comparing severe AFMR opposed severe DMR and preserved LVEF (mean EROA 0.44 ± 0.18 cm^2 vs 0.53 ± 0.11 cm^2, respectively), with AFMR independently linked to mortality (adjusted OR 2.6). Naturally, all-cause mortality rates were substantially higher relative to age and gender-matched controls, peaking up to 50% at 5 year-follow up in the Olmsted County community study[9] (**Fig. 9**). The proportion of HFpEF (and thereby its relative weight on outcomes) in the abovementioned epidemiological studies is unknown but presumed to be substantial. Presumably, a group of HFpEF lacking significant AFMR might have served as a better comparator, given many questions remain about the relative impact of this low-volume MR as opposed to HFpEF with LA myopathy on outcomes.

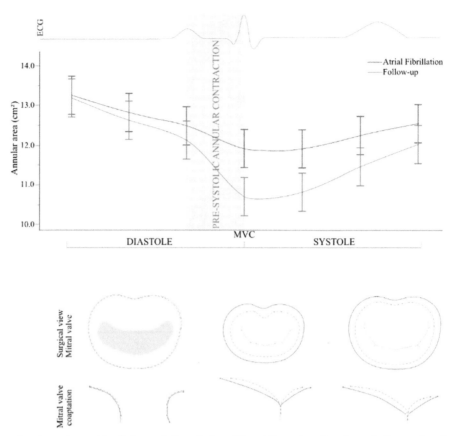

Fig. 6. Annular dynamics and leaflet coaptation during AF and 6 weeks after sinus rhythm restoration. Mitral annular dynamics are impaired during persistent AF, particularly during pre-systole. Regained pre-systolic annular contraction improves leaflet coaptation throughout systole which benefits AFMR severity, irrespective of LA shrinkage. AF, atrial fibrillation; LA, left atrial; MR, mitral regurgitation; MV, mitral valve; MVC, mitral valve closure. (*Adapted from* Deferm S, Bertrand PB, Verhaert D, et al. Mitral Annular Dynamics in AF versus Sinus Rhythm: Novel Insights Into the Mechanism of AFMR. JACC Cardiovasc Imaging. 2022;15(1):1-13.)

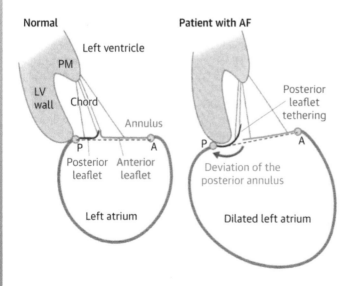

Fig. 7. Mechanism of eccentric jet in AFMR. The posterior MA is anchored between the LA and the crest of the LV inlet. In giant LA, the posterior part of the MA is pulled toward the epicardial surface of the basal posterior LV wall. The posterior leaflet is pulled along with it, thereby increasing the normal annulo-papillary distance. This so-called "atriogenic posterior leaflet tethering" inflicts an eccentric AFMR jet. (*From* Kagiyama N, Mondillo S, Yoshida K, Mandoli GE, Cameli M. Subtypes of Atrial Functional Mitral Regurgitation: Imaging Insights Into Their Mechanisms and Therapeutic Implications. JACC Cardiovasc Imaging. 2020;13(3):820-835.)

HFpEF

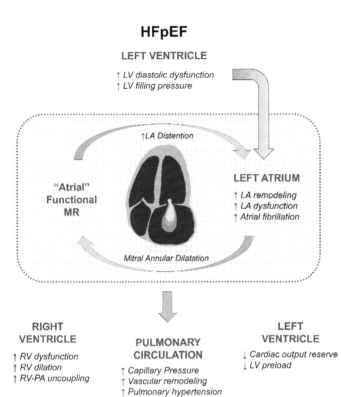

LEFT VENTRICLE
↑ *LV diastolic dysfunction*
↑ *LV filling pressure*

↑*LA Distention*

"Atrial"
Functional
MR

LEFT ATRIUM
↑ *LA remodeling*
↑ *LA dysfunction*
↑ *Atrial fibrillation*

Mitral Annular Dilatation

Fig. 8. Pathogenesis of AFMR, LA myopathy and their relation in HFpEF. AFMR, atrial functional mitral regurgitation; HFpEF, heart failure with preserved ejection fraction; LA, left atrium/atrial; LV, left ventricle/ventricular; PA, pulmonary artery/arterial; RV, right ventricle/ventricular. (*From* Tamargo M, Obokata M, Reddy YNV, et al. Functional mitral regurgitation and left atrial myopathy in heart failure with preserved ejection fraction. *Eur J Heart Fail*. 2020;22(3):489-498.)

RIGHT VENTRICLE
↑ *RV dysfunction*
↑ *RV dilation*
↑ *RV-PA uncoupling*

PULMONARY CIRCULATION
↑ *Capillary Pressure*
↑ *Vascular remodeling*
↑ *Pulmonary hypertension*

LEFT VENTRICLE
↓ *Cardiac output reserve*
↓ *LV preload*

Moderate-to-severe functional MR was reported in 20% of HFpEF cases in the prospective european society of cardiology, heart failure (ESC HF) registry.[37] In addition, the ATTEND (Acute Decompensated Heart Failure Syndromes)—registry learned that mild or worse functional MR at discharge remained highly prevalent in 1800 individuals with acutely decompensated HFpEF.[38] Even when mild, any MR at discharge significantly impacted all-cause mortality and

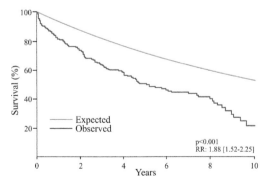

Fig. 9. All-cause mortality in AFMR, opposed to expected survival in age- and sex-matched controls. RR, relative risk. (*From* Dziadzko V, Dziadzko M, Medina-Inojosa JR, et al. Causes and mechanisms of isolated mitral regurgitation in the community: clinical context and outcome. Eur Heart J. 2019;40(27):2194-2202.)

heart failure rehospitalizations (adjusted hazard ratio [HR] 1.40).

In conclusion, both AFMR and HFpEF, as well as their coexistence have been linked to adverse outcomes. At present, this type of MR remains a conundrum. Further study is highly needed to unravel the chain of causality between moderate-to-worse AFMR, LA myopathy, and outcomes. Although the high burden of comorbidities in AFMR impacts prognosis, it is plausible that this low-volume MR poses a significant stress for a non-dilated noncompliant LV and LA with restrictive physiology (paralleling the disproportionality concept such as in ventricular functional MR).[7] Equally important, whether poor outcomes are driven by AFMR itself or rather the underlying LA myopathy in HFpEF is unknown, given their frequent coexistence. Differently put, whether AFMR should be regarded as a risk marker or rather a risk factor for poor outcomes, is to be answered.[34] A prospective trial randomizing HFpEF with significant AMFR for a therapeutic intervention versus optimal medical therapy, might partially unravel this enigma.[7]

EVALUATION OF ATRIAL FUNCTIONAL MITRAL REGURGITATION

From the abovementioned mechanisms (see section on Nature of the Problem), one may conclude that normal LV size and sphericity, preserved LVEF, and LA plus MA dilation are the key echocardiographic features in AFMR[6,7,12] (see **Fig. 2**). The mitral valve leaflets are considered structurally normal, although mild fibrotic leaflet thickening or annular calcification can be seen.[6] Reduced LV global longitudinal strain and LV hypertrophy may be present, especially in those with concomitant HFpEF. Moderate-to-severe biatrial and annular dilation are typically observed, with a systolic anteroposterior diameter greater than 35 mm (measured in parasternal long axis) indicating MA dilation.[6,7,39] Presumably, three dimensional (3D) echocardiographic measurements of annular area will become standard practice, given slightly better correlation with computed tomography (CT).[40]

Importantly, the echocardiographic distinction between AFMR and VFMR should not uniquely rely on chamber/annular measurements, as longstanding volume overload equally causes atrial and annular dilation in VFMR. The characteristic that most differentiates AFMR from the VFMR is the level of leaflet coaptation. Subvalvular leaflet tethering in VFMR shifts the coaptation point away from the annular plane toward the LV apex inflicting an eccentric or central jet depending on asymmetric or symmetric tethering, respectively. The classic "seagull sign" may point to substantial anterior subvalvular leaflet tethering in this case. In contrast, in AFMR, the leaflets remain confined to the annular plane with a central regurgitant jet dispersed across the entire coaptation line.[6,12] A mild degree of tenting is often visualized as the mitral valve leaflets lose their concavity toward the LV apex (ie, flatten) in their attempt to compensate for annular enlargement.[19] As annular dilation progresses and the height of the posterior leaflet decreases, the AFMR-jet is more likely to become eccentric (ie, in the process of "atriogenic posterior leaflet tethering," see **Fig. 7**).[18,27,41] Both AFMR and VFMR can be seen as two opposite ends of the "functional MR-spectrum" which by itself shows considerable overlap. This is corroborated by a recent subanalysis from the COAPT study (Cardiovascular Outcomes Assessment of the MitraClip Percutaneous Therapy for Heart Failure Patients with Functional Mitral Regurgitation) which showed that patients with VFMR and a history of AF had smaller LV volumes but larger LA and mitral valve EROA, suggesting an important atrial component on the top of VFMR.[42] Viceversa, long-standing volume overload in AFMR may adversely affect LV size and function.

An integrated approach using a combination of qualitative, semi-quantitative, and quantitative parameters is used to grade MR-severity (each of which has its own constraints).[43] The proximal convergence method may underestimate the EROA, as the regurgitant jet usually extends across the coaptation line resulting in an elliptical orifice shape.[6,7] In addition, the temporal patterns of mitral regurgitant flow and orifice area variation are often neglected.[44] Measuring the 3D vena contracta area may overcome flow and geometric assumptions, but yet has to find widespread acceptance in daily clinical practice.[45,46] A blunted systolic pulmonary vein inflow can simply result from AF or LA myopathy, even in the absence of significant AFMR.

Furthermore, the assessment of MR severity is troubled by AF itself, particularly in those with rapid or very irregular rhythms. Consequently, the timing of echocardiographic assessment seems important, in the knowledge that many show marked improvement in severity following sinus rhythm restoration.[13,26] It is recommended to assess severity either during stable sinus rhythm, or otherwise, in AF with well-controlled ventricular pace using the indexed beat method (ie, selection of a beat with equal preceding and pre-preceding interval).[7,47] In addition, the currently used quantitative thresholds to define disease severity are derived from studies VFMR and therefore have not been validated in AFMR.[7,12,48] Aside from the discussion whether prognosis in AFMR is governed by LA myopathy or AFMR itself,[34] it may be plausible that a lower regurgitant volume is yet hemodynamically significant in subjects with "stiff," restrictive physiology (alluding to the disproportionality concept, as historically discussed in VFMR[49,50]).

CT and cardiac magnetic resonance imaging (CMR) allows for a detailed structural analysis of the mitral valve morphology, annular size,[41,51] and geometrical changes of the MA throughout the cardiac cycle. CMR can reliably assess MR-severity through volumetric measurements[52] while offering a more comprehensive assessment of LV remodeling.[53] Furthermore, delayed enhancement CMR may provide insights into the severity and etiology of the underlying cardiomyopathy. Although its use in the context of AFMR is limited, the extent of atrial fibrosis has been linked to arrhythmia recurrence and procedural success following catheter ablation of AF.[41,54,55]

THERAPEUTIC OPTIONS FOR ATRIAL FUNCTIONAL MITRAL REGURGITATION

The management of AFMR is mostly based on expert opinion, given the paucity of data and the fact that AFMR is only now truthfully acknowledged as a distinct entity by the guidelines.[56,57]

Based on the current data, AFMR management is based on rhythm control strategies, optimal medical therapy, and therapeutic interventions when applicable.

Rhythm Control Strategies

Multiple studies have claimed a significant reduction in AFMR severity in those with successful sinus rhythm maintenance following pulmonary vein isolation[13,58] or electrical cardioversion.[26,59] This reduction has been attributed to favorable LA and MA remodeling which benefits leaflet coaptation and thus AFMR. For instance, in one of the very first studies by Gertz and colleagues,[13] 82% of patients with AF recurrence still showed significant AFMR, as opposed to only 24% of successfully ablated patients (see **Fig. 3**). Furthermore, sinus rhythm restoration allows for a gradual recovery of presystolic annular dynamics which improves leaflet apposition and thus annular-leaflet imbalance, regardless of global LA remodeling[26] (see **Fig. 6**). These studies provide a compelling case to strive for a rhythm control strategy and are further supported by the recently published Early Rhythm-Control Therapy in Patients with Atrial Fibrillation study.[60] The latter trial was stopped prematurely after showing far less cardiovascular mortality and HF hospitalizations in those with early AF with cardiovascular conditions randomized for rhythm control versus usual care. This effect was consistent across those with and without preexistent heart failure. Furthermore, rhythm control strategies have been linked to decreases in circulating brain natriuretic peptides and increases in LVEF,[60,61] which may indirectly benefit AFMR.

Optimal Medical Therapy

Beyond rhythm control therapy, few data exist on the efficacy of optimal medical therapy in the management of AFMR. Theoretically, medical therapy intended to lower atrial pressure overload in HFpEF could cease a vicious cycle of unfavorable atrial remodeling and fibrosis, potential AF, and thus AFMR.[12,62] Although disease-modifying therapy exists for heart failure with reduced ejection fraction (HFrEF), few such options are known to be effective in heart failure with higher range of LVEF.[63] Inhibition of the renin-angiotensin-aldosteron axis by Candesartan only slightly reduced AF incidence in HFpEF by interfering with the fibrotic atrial remodeling process.[64] Two recent studies[65,66] claimed significant reductions in MR severity, along large reductions in N-terminal pro-B-natriuretic peptide and reverse cardiac remodeling in HFrEF randomized for treatment with sacubitril–valsartan. Whether these results are partially extrapolatable to HFpEF with AFMR is unclear. Hence, sacubitril–valsartan did not significantly lower rate the rate of heart failure hospitalizations and cardiovascular death in HFpEF[67] as opposed to HFrEF.[68] Further subanalysis, however, found that its therapeutic benefits may extend to a higher LVEF range in women.[63] At cellular/molecular level, sacubitril–valsartan inhibits degradation of natriuretic peptides and tissue-growth facture beta (TGFβ), which, respectively, may promote natriuresis[69] and prevent leaflet fibrosis without interfering with leaflet growth.[24] Theoretically, both effects could prove beneficial for AFMR-reduction by reducing LA volumes, pressures and optimizing the ongoing annular-leaflet imbalance. Finally, both empagliflozin[70] and dapagliflozin[71] were first to successfully lower the risk of cardiovascular death and worsening heart failure in HFpEF, with no difference in benefit regardless the presence of type 2 diabetes mellitus nor atrial arrhythmias at enrollment. Also, its class effect seems very promising for lowering LA stresses and AF-prevalence.[72]

Mitral Valve Surgery

Data on the surgical management of AFMR remain limited. Based on expert consensus and the current limited level of evidence (C), the 2020 American college of cardioloige/American heart association (ACC/AHA) guidelines[56] offer a class IIb indication ("may be considered") for surgery in subjects with severe AFMR who remain symptomatic in spite optimal medical therapy.

Mitral valve surgery most commonly involves surgical ring annuloplasty which can improve leaflet coaptation and therefore MR, by decreasing the antero-posterior annular dimension. Surgical interventions targeting the mitral valve have yielded controversial results in VFMR. Short-term observational data showed significant reverse LV remodeling[73] and improvements in LV systolic function.[74] Nevertheless, persisting subvalvular leaflet tethering[75] leading to MR-recurrence[76,77] or functional mitral stenosis,[78,79] together with the lack of survival benefit,[80–82] have led to a less common use of surgical annuloplasty in VFMR. In contrast, two recent retrospective cohort studies[83,84] found surgical annuloplasty can provide a durable MR reduction and better overall outcomes when annular-leaflet imbalance is the predominant mechanism for leaflet malcoaptation (Carpentier I MR, AFMR), as opposed to VFMR with subvalvular leaflet tethering (Carpentier IIIb MR). This superiority for surgical annuloplasty in AFMR was apparent even when corrected for all-cause mortality as competing risk and major differences in baseline risk profile.[83]

In those with giant left atria and possible posterior "atriogenic" leaflet tethering, extreme restrictive annuloplasty is to be avoided given the risk of ring dehiscence. Mitral valve implantation could provide an alternative in selective cases, with attendance to avoid LV outflow tract obstruction in small cavities. Posterior leaflet augmentation with an autologous pericardial patch has been advocated by some,[85] albeit with the risk of future leaflet stiffening.

Currently, the position of surgical repair in the landscape of AFMR remains uncertain. Surgical annuloplasty could serve as a bail-out therapy when rhythm-control strategies and optimal medical therapy fail to reverse severe AFMR.[83] However, given the advent of newer TEER devices resulting in more extensive valve repair, as well as the risk profile of many AFMR-subject with various comorbidities, TEER is likely to be the first preferable option in this scenario.

Transcatheter Treatment

Four studies recently explored the safety and efficacy of TEER in AFMR,[86–89] as compared with either DMR or VFMR, or both. Most differences in-between studies largely relate to different used cutoffs for LV/LA dimensions and, more importantly, slight variations in the definition of AFMR (eg, Sodhi and colleagues[87] only included patients with a history of AF, whereas in other studies previous AF was not a prerequisite). Depending on the applied definition, AFMR constituted 5% to 10% of TEER cases, phenotypically differing from DMR and VFMR. Overall, TEER provided a sustained MR reduction in AFMR with equal[87,89] or slightly lower[86] mortality and adverse events rates at 1 to 2-year follow-up, as opposed to VFMR. Unsurprisingly, preoperative NYHA class and right ventricular (RV) dysfunction were linked to post-TEER survival in AFMR.[89] Procedural success rates were markedly lower (74.1% in AFMR) in the study by Tanaka and colleagues,[88] and presumably ascribed to the use of a more stringent criterion for procedural success (MR reduction ≤1+) as well as the use of older generation Mitra-Clip devices (Abbott Vascular) with suboptimal MR reduction. The current fourth generation Mitra-Clip (Abbott Vascular) XTW and NTW devices (Abbott Vascular) offers a broadened coaptation area which is expected to result in a more extensive valve repair. This design optimization may become particularly important in AFMR with large annular-leaflet imbalance, as evidenced by a 95% procedural success rate in AFMR treated with fourth-generation devices in the same study.[88] In addition, the immediate reduction in anteroposterior diameter and thus MA area by TEER adds to procedural success.[90,91]

NATURE OF THE PROBLEM IN ATRIAL FUNCTIONAL MITRAL REGURGITATION

With the increased recognition of "isolated or idiopathic" TR in daily clinical practice, the number of papers devoted to its clinical impact, prognosis, and mechanisms of disease has grown substantially (**Fig. 10**). In that aspect, caution should be taken for its inhomogeneous definition in literature.[92] For some, it is defined as TR which occurs "in isolation," that is to say without the presence of other significant valve disease. Others, however, refer to it as TR which is neither of primary nor secondary origin, but instead develops due to right atrial (RA) dilation, so-called AFTR.[93] To avoid any confusion, the term "AFTR" instead of "isolated/idiopathic TR" shall be used throughout the remaining article wherever appropriate.

AFTR and AFMR are two manifestations of the same disease. This implies that the same stimuli responsible for LA and annular dilation in AFMR also affect the RA and tricuspid annulus (TA). More so, compared with its left-sided counterpart, the normal annulus is larger (7.6 ± 1.7 cm/m² in mid-systole) and mainly composed of fat making it more predisposed to dilate which in turn explains the remarkably high prevalence of concomitant TR in the AFMR population. Most evidence stems from studies observing significant TR in elderly subjects with long-standing AF in the absence of RV dilation or dysfunction and therefore formerly coined "idiopathic or isolated."[16,94–98] These cases contrasted with secondary TR in the setting of left heart disease through larger annular size which correlated closely with RA area[16] rather than RV end-diastolic volume.[95]

Of note, "any TR begets TR," referring to a vicious circle in which the ongoing volume overload in any TR causes progressive RV dysfunction, increased subvalvular tethering, and therefore increasing TR. This also implies that ongoing volume load by AFTR—while initially accompanied grounded on annular dilation with no or only mild RV dysfunction—may eventually cause substantial RV dysfunction with subvalvular tethering.

EPIDEMIOLOGY AND CLINICAL OUTCOMES OF ATRIAL FUNCTIONAL MITRAL REGURGITATION

Regardless of the underlying etiological subgroup, isolated TR (of any cause) significantly impacts

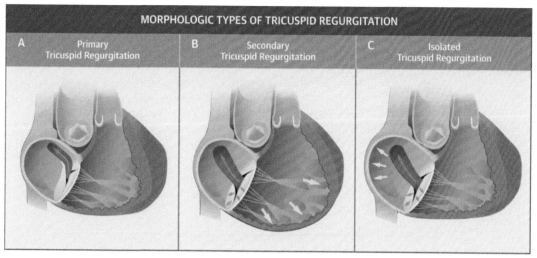

Fig. 10. Morphological types of tricuspid regurgitation. Primary TR refers to TR caused by an intrinsic defect of the tricuspid valve apparatus. In secondary TR, a coaptation gap occurs due to RV dilation/dysfunction which leads to significant subvalvular leaflet tethering. These days, so-called "isolated TR" is increasingly recognized, with dilation of the tricuspid annulus and right atrium in the context of AF. Care should be taken with the imprecise definition of "isolated TR" in literature (see full text). (*A*) primary tricuspid regurgitation; (*B*) secondary 'ventricular functional' tricuspid regurgitation; (*C*) isolated tricuspid regurgitation due to atrial and annular dilation or atrial functional tricuspid regurgitation. (*From* Prihadi EA, Delgado V, Leon MB, Enriquez-Sarano M, Topilsky Y, Bax JJ. Morphologic Types of Tricuspid Regurgitation: Characteristics and Prognostic Implications. JACC Cardiovasc Imaging. 2019;12(3):491-499.)

morbidity and mortality, either independently or through progression of RV dysfunction.[99–104] In the largest contemporary cohort focused on clinically significant isolated TR (ie, TR in isolation, $n = 9045$),[102] approximately 95% of cases were of functional origin. Of these, over one-half stemmed from secondary TR in the setting of left-sided heart disease (54.4%) followed by AFTR (24.3%) and cor pulmonale (17%). AFTR patients matched the typical phenotype of an elderly predominant female patient with a high burden of comorbidities and nearly 90% prevalence rate of AF. Unsurprisingly, outcomes in TR secondary to left-sided heart or pulmonary disease were significantly worse as compared with AFTR (**Fig. 11**). Of note, the proposed 16-point risk score model for all-cause mortality may be less useable in early stages of AFTR (without RV dysfunction) given the weight penalty of RV dysfunction on mortality.

Currently, few conclusive data exist on the natural progression of TR in patients with new-onset AF. In a population-based cohort of subjects with new-onset AF lacking left-sided heart disease or significant valvular heart disease at baseline ($n = 691$), nearly one-third developed moderate or greater TR of any cause over a median follow-up of 13.3 years.[105] Of these, 32% (10.6% of the entire cohort) were deemed AFTR corresponding to an incidence rate of 1.3 cases per 100 person-years. Female sex, age, and persistent/permanent

AF with rate control were independent predictors for any TR progression while handling all-cause death as competing risk. In line with previous data, the development of significant TR of any cause and AFTR significantly impacted mortality (adjusted HR resp. 2.92 and 1.51, **Fig. 12**).

EVALUATION OF ATRIAL FUNCTIONAL MITRAL REGURGITATION

Two-dimensional and 3D echocardiography are first-line image modalities for a thorough evaluation of the tricuspid valve apparatus, RA size, RV size, and function while assessing the underlying mechanism and severity of TR.

Secondary TR in the setting of RV pressure overload (left-sided heart disease or marked pulmonary hypertension) leads to a spherical deformation of the RV with RA and TA dilation being a consequence of long-standing TR rather than an initiator. This disproportionate RV apical remodeling response typically causes substantial leaflet tethering with either an eccentric or central jet (eg, the coaptation point is displayed from the annular plane toward the apex).[93,95,96,106] In contrast, in AFTR, the leaflets appear flattened and confined to the annular plane. The RV retains its conical shape though mild dilation of the basal inflow region may appear in response to overt annular dilation.[106–108] The central jet originates

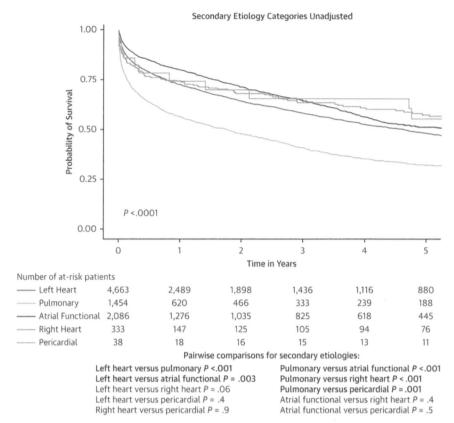

Fig. 11. Kaplan–Meier survival curves according to functional/secondary TR etiology (unadjusted for confounders). Survival in AFTR was significantly better as compared with secondary TR in the setting of left heart and pulmonary disease. (*From* Wang TKM, Akyuz K, Mentias A, et al. Contemporary Etiologies, Outcomes, and Novel Risk Score for Isolated Tricuspid Regurgitation. *JACC Cardiovasc Imaging.* 2022;15(5):731-744.)

slightly more posteroseptal as annular enlargement particularly affects the fat-rich posteroseptal part[95,96,108] (**Figs. 13** and **14**).

Current guidelines[43] advocate an integrated approach based on a structural assessment and a combination of qualitative, semi-quantitative, and quantitative parameters to define disease severity. Each of these parameters has its own relative utility and set of limitations,[109,110] regardless the underlying etiological phenotype (similar to AFMR). In addition, it is believed in terms of prognosis that "not all severe TR is the same." Indeed, regurgitant volumes are typically much higher as seen in the mitral space. Especially in this era of transcatheter therapy, a revised grading scheme including "massive" and "torrential" TR has been proposed supporting the belief that any TR reduction may be associated with a decrease in mortality.[111] Currently, all major trials have used this new grading scheme, even though it is not inherited in current guidelines. In addition, a new leaflet nomenclature was recently introduced given the growing recognition of variability in

leaflet morphology which likely contributes to the procedural success of transcatheter therapy.[112] A detailed discussion on RV assessment in severe TR falls outside the scope of this article. Although RV function is usually preserved in early stages of AFTR, one should bear in mind that the RV dysfunction can be masked by the unloading effect of severe TR. Noninvasive markers of RV-pulmonary arterial coupling may overcome this limitation.[113]

CMR is still considered the gold standard for RV assessment given its excellent spatial resolution without restrictions related to body size, acoustic windows, and radiation.[114,115] In addition, it allows for additional insights in the pattern of myocardial fibrosis and TR-severity, respectively, by late gadolinium enhancement imaging and volumetric subtractions.[7] Pre-procedural cardiac CT is the key for patient selection when considering transcatheter tricuspid valve replacement or repair techniques targeting the TA.[116,117] It provides valuable information of the tricuspid apparatus morphology, anchoring sites, vascular access,

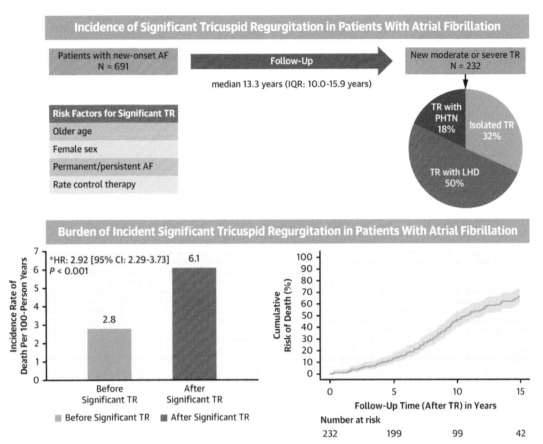

Fig. 12. Incidence and burden of significant TR in patients with new-onset AF. Nearly one-third with new-onset AF developed significant TR after a median follow-up of 13.3 years. Isolated TR comprised one-third of these cases and adversely impacted mortality rates. AF, atrial fibrillation; HR, hazard ratio; IQR, interquartile ranges; TR, tricuspid regurgitation. (*From* Patlolla SH, Schaff HV, Nishimura RA, et al. Incidence and Burden of Tricuspid Regurgitation in Patients With Atrial Fibrillation. *J Am Coll Cardiol.* 2022;80(24):2289-2298.)

and most importantly the anatomical relationship to key surrounding structures such as the right coronary artery.

THERAPEUTIC OPTIONS FOR ATRIAL FUNCTIONAL MITRAL REGURGITATION
Rhythm Control Strategies

As for the mitral valve, several authors advocated a rhythm control strategy in light of reducing AFTR through beneficial RA reverse remodeling.[98,100] The impact of cardiac chamber remodeling on functional regurgitation was yet again established in 117 patients hospitalized for AF.[118] At 12-month follow-up, only those with active restoration of sinus rhythm (n = 47, either through cardioversion or ablation) without relapse showed a manifest decrease in chamber volumes and functional improvement. Although data on AF burden were lacking, AFTR significantly improved in patients with successful rhythm "maintenance"

at 12 month-follow up (either following spontaneous or active sinus rhythm restoration). These findings are further complemented by data from Patlolla and colleagues[105] studying the incidence and burden of TR in patients with new-onset AF. One-third developed significant TR of any cause (of which 32% were deemed AFTR) which conferred significant mortality risk. Importantly, a rhythm control strategy was independently associated with lower risk of developing TR.

Optimal Medical Therapy

There is limited proof that medical therapy significantly affects outcome, despite its ability to lower symptoms in a subset of isolated TR. Theoretically, drug therapy focused at lowering atrial pressures has the potential to break the vicious circle of negative atrial remodeling, fibrosis, and atrial functional regurgitation.[12] In that aspect, the class effect of the above-mentioned drugs in the section on

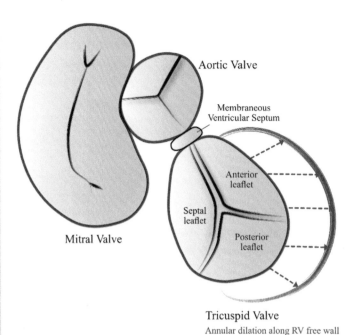

Aortic Valve

Membraneous
Ventricular Septum

Anterior
leaflet

Septal
leaflet

Posterior
leaflet

Mitral Valve

Tricuspid Valve

Annular dilation along RV free wall

Fig. 13. The tricuspid annulus with its anatomic relations. Tricuspid annular dilation primarily affects the lateral part along the RV free wall. RV, right ventricular. (*From* Silbiger JJ. Atrial functional tricuspid regurgitation: An underappreciated cause of secondary tricuspid regurgitation. *Echocardiography.* 2019;36(5):954-957.)

AFMR may also benefit AFTR either directly or indirectly. In the same light, diuretics may effectively treat episodes of volume overload and prevent further worsening of AFTR (as "TR begets TR").[100]

Tricuspid Valve Surgery

Current guidelines[56,57] mainly cover TR management in the setting of concomitant left-side valvular surgery, rather than isolated TR or AFTR given the scarcity of data.[92] Moreover, existing recommendations for isolated TR are based on data in young patients with primary tricuspid valve flail.[100] Obviously, this group is fundamentally different from AFTR affecting an elderly patient with AF and many comorbidities.

Thus, even though isolated TR and AFTR are prevalent and associated with ominous outcome,[99,101] both remain markedly undertreated as compared with left-sided valvular disease.[119,120] The rarity of surgery for isolated TR can be traced to the inability of consistently proving a survival benefit in several registries,[120–122] at the cost of high perioperative mortality up to 10%.[121,123] Furthermore, Axtell and colleagues[124] found no survival benefit of surgery beyond medical management in a small propensity matched sample of isolated TR. No data on RV dysfunction, right heart invasive measurements or AF prevalence were available, which therefore implies that the study results cannot simply be extrapolated to AFTR.

In addition, delayed surgical referral may adversely impact outcomes by allowing for the development of RV dysfunction and end-organ

failure.[100,105] Unlike with left-sided valvular disease, no data are available to guide the appropriate timing of surgery in isolated TR. One recent study by the Mayo group reported better perioperative and postoperative outcomes following timely performed surgery in isolated TR, before the development of significant RV dysfunction.[125] This topic may become particularly relevant in subjects with AFTR who often show less RV dysfunction initially, as compared with secondary TR.[102] However, as time fades by the ensuing volume load may initiate a vicious circle in which TR begets TR by worsening RV function.

Even more importantly, the above-mentioned studies should be interpreted cautiously considering all of them focused on a very heterogeneous group of "TR in isolation," instead of AFTR. Improved etiology adjudication and risk stratification are much needed in isolated TR before exposing the patient to any intervention, especially in the era of transcatheter therapy.[92]

Transcatheter Treatment

The advent of minimally invasive transcatheter tricuspid therapy provides a valuable alternative to treat isolated TR, particularly in those at high surgical risk without response to medical therapy. Current transcatheter repair options mimic surgical techniques and improve coaptation either directly by acting on the leaflets (TEER) or indirectly by acting on the annulus (annuloplasty and annular cinching devices). The most widely applied

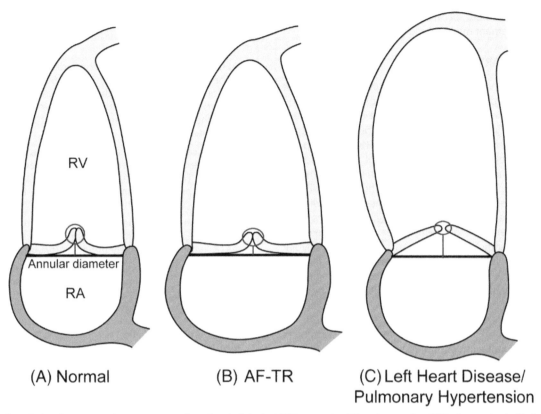

Fig. 14. Leaflet coaptation patterns and tenting height in AFTR versus traditional secondary TR in the context of left-sided heart disease or pulmonary hypertension. In AFTR, excessive annular dilation pulls the leaflets apart without significantly altering tenting height (can be mildly reduced). Mild basal RV dilation may appear, though the overall shape of the RV is maintained. In contrast, in secondary TR in the setting of left heart or pulmonary disease annular dilation is less prominent but tenting height is increased due to leaflet tethering. AFTR, atrial functional tricuspid regurgitation; RA, right atrium; RV, right ventricle. (A) coaptation pattern in absence of tricuspid regurgitation; (B) coaptation pattern in the context of atrial functional tricuspid regurgitation; (C) coaptation pattern in the context of ventricular functional tricuspid regurgitation. (*From* Silbiger JJ. Atrial functional tricuspid regurgitation: An underappreciated cause of secondary tricuspid regurgitation. *Echocardiography.* 2019;36(5):954-957.)

technique to treat TR of any cause is TEER, which has shown to effectively reduce TR, improve symptoms and prompt significant reverse RV remodeling.[126] The TRILUMINATE study (Trial to Evaluate Treatment with Abbott Transcatheter Clip Repair System in Patients with Moderate or Greater Tricuspid Regurgitation) reported relatively low 1-year mortality (7.1%) besides moderate or less TR in 71% of cases 1 year following treatment with the Triclip NT device. Similarly, 52% of patients experienced moderate TR or less with no mortality 30 days after treatment with the Pascal device (CLASP TR study, Edwards PASCAL Transcatheter Valve Repair System in Tricuspid Regurgitation).[127] In these early feasibility trials, approximately 90% of cases had a history of AF, though the distinct phenotypes of TR were not identified in spite their known impact on outcomes.[128] Thus, studies comparing hard endpoints following transcatheter

treatment versus optimal medical therapy in TR and by extension AFTR are eagerly awaited. Enrollment in the TRILUMINATE Pivotal trial (NCT03904147, comparison of Triclip versus optimal medical therapy in symptomatic patients with severe TR, who are at intermediate or greater estimated risk for mortality or morbidity with tricuspid valve surgery) is currently completed. In anticipation of these results, the multi-device TriValve registry claimed lower mortality and heart failure hospitalizations following transcatheter tricuspid valve therapy in TR of any cause compared with using propensity-matched analysis. TEER constituted 55% of these interventions. Nowadays, the armamentarium is expanding with large coaptation gaps now being treated with the newest generation TriClip, which also adds the possibility for independent leaflet grasping. In those with a coaptation gap greater than 10 mm,[129] off-label use of transcatheter tricuspid valve replacement might provide a safety net.[116,130]

SUMMARY

AFMR and AFTR are increasingly observed in our greying population with a high burden of AF and comorbidities. These forms of functional atrioventricular valve regurgitation are grounded on atrial/annular dilation plus dysfunction. Key in their pathophysiology is the concept of annular-leaflet imbalance, in which leaflet growth fails to compensate for excessive annular dilation, often with the occurrence of a central regurgitant jet. Owing to this peculiar pathophysiology, prognosis and treatment options vastly differ as compared with their ventricular counterpart in which subvalvular leaflet tethering is the predominant feature. AFMR is linked to poor prognosis as compared with controls and DMR in spite often being a low-volume MR. Similarly, nearly one in three patients with new-onset AF develops isolated TR, of which AFTR comprises one in three cases and significantly impacts prognosis. Based on current evidence, management consists of optimal medical therapy and rhythm control strategies, with therapeutic interventions in those where sinus rhythm restoration is either not feasible or does not lead to a favorable reduction in atrioventricular valve regurgitation. Currently, most evidence exists for the treatment of AFMR, with recent efficacy trials demonstrating high procedural success rates following TEER.

CLINICS CARE POINTS

- With the projected shift to an older population with a high burden of atrial fibrillation (AF) and heart failure with preserved ejection fraction, it is expected that the frequency of atrial functional mitral and tricuspid regurgitation (AFMR and AFTR) will increase accordingly.
- The distinction between atrioventricular valve regurgitation in the context of ventricular versus. atrial disease is crucial, given their different pathophysiologic backgrounds and treatment needs.
- Both AFMR and AFTR are manifestations of the same disease in which *annular-leaflet imbalance (failure of the leaflets to match excessive annular dilation)* hampers normal leaflet coaptation. Tenting height is most often preserved or only slightly affected, as opposed to mitral regurgitation/tricuspid regurgitation (MR/TR) in the setting of ventricular disease.

- Recent efficacy trials show good procedural results of transcatheter edge-to-edge repair in the setting of AFMR.
- AFMR remains a clinical conundrum with poor prognosis. It is unclear if poor outcomes are primarily driven by the high burden of comorbidities, the underlying LA myopathy or rather the AFMR itself. Further study is warranted (see above).
- Specific care should be attained to the rather imprecise term "isolated TR" which is used to refer to TR "in isolation" versus TR that is neither primary/secondary of origin but caused by excessive annular dilation.
- Nearly one-third of patients with new-onset AF develop significant TR, of which 32% are AFTR, which significantly impacts mortality.
- "TR begets TR." The ensuing volume load in TR instigates a vicious circle with adverse right ventricular (RV) remodeling, increased subvalvular tethering and worsening TR. The same mechanism could theoretically cause AFTR (initially without major RV dysfunction) to deteriorate due to an additional ventricular component when RV dysfunction eventually occurs.
- Even though isolated TR is associated with ominous outcomes, it remains markedly undertreated due to high mortality rates in previous surgical registries.
- With the advent of transcatheter therapy, severe TR has come into the therapeutic radar. Especially in this era, careful etiology adjudication is crucial based on a combination of clinical and echocardiographic parameters, possibly augmented by other imaging modalities. The critical question remains "who to treat" and "when exactly to treat."

DISCLOSURES

Dr R.S. Von Bardeleben has received consultancy fees from Edwards Lifesciences, Abbott Laboratory and Medtronic. Other authors have nothing to declare with relation to this article.

FUNDING

Dr S. Deferm has been funded by the ERASMUS+ grant (outgoing international mobility).

REFERENCES

1. Chugh SS, Havmoeller R, Narayanan K, et al. Worldwide epidemiology of atrial fibrillation: A global burden of disease 2010 study. Circulation 2014;129(8):837–47.

2. Go AS, Hylek EM, Phillips KA, et al. Prevalence of Diagnosed Atrial Fibrillation in Adults. JAMA 2001;285(18):2370.

3. Benjamin EJ, Muntner P, Alonso A, et al. Heart Disease and Stroke Statistics-2019 Update: A Report From the American Heart Association. Circulation 2019;139(10). https://doi.org/10.1161/CIR.000000 0000000659.

4. Colilla S, Crow A, Petkun W, et al. Estimates of current and future incidence and prevalence of atrial fibrillation in the U.S. adult population. Am J Cardiol 2013;112(8):1142–7.

5. Kornej J, Börschel CS, Benjamin EJ, et al. Epidemiology of Atrial Fibrillation in the 21st Century Novel Methods and New Insights. Circ Res 2020;127:4–20.

6. Deferm S, Bertrand PB, Verbrugge FH, et al. Atrial Functional Mitral Regurgitation. J Am Coll Cardiol 2019;73(19):2465–76.

7. Zoghbi WA, Levine RA, Flachskampf F, et al. Atrial Functional Mitral Regurgitation. JACC Cardiovasc Imaging 2022;15(11):1870–82.

8. Mesi O, Gad MM, Crane AD, et al. Severe Atrial Functional Mitral Regurgitation: Clinical and Echocardiographic Characteristics, Management and Outcomes. JACC Cardiovasc Imaging 2021;14(4): 797–808.

9. Dziadzko V, Dziadzko M, Medina-Inojosa JR, et al. Causes and mechanisms of isolated mitral regurgitation in the community: Clinical context and outcome. Eur Heart J 2019;40(27):2194–202.

10. Asgar AW, Mack MJ, Stone GW. Secondary mitral regurgitation in heart failure: Pathophysiology, prognosis, and therapeutic considerations. J Am Coll Cardiol 2015;65(12):1231–48.

11. Bertrand PB, Schwammenthal E, Levine RA, et al. Exercise Dynamics in Secondary Mitral Regurgitation: Pathophysiology and Therapeutic Implications. Circulation 2017;135(3):297–314.

12. Deferm S, Dauw J, Vandervoort PM, et al. Atrial Functional Mitral and Tricuspid Regurgitation. Curr Treat Options Cardiovasc Med 2020;22(10):30.

13. Gertz ZM, Raina A, Saghy L, et al. Evidence of Atrial Functional Mitral Regurgitation Due to Atrial Fibrillation. J Am Coll Cardiol 2011;58(14):1474–81.

14. Yap J, Bolling SF, Rogers JH. Contemporary Review in Interventional Cardiology: Mitral Annuloplasty in Secondary Mitral Regurgitation. Struct Heart 2021; 1–16. https://doi.org/10.1080/24748706.2021.189 5457.

15. Otsuji Y, Kumanohoso T, Yoshifuku S, et al. Isolated annular dilation does not usually cause important functional mitral regurgitation: Comparison between patients with lone atrial fibrillation and those with idiopathic or ischemic cardiomyopathy. J Am Coll Cardiol 2002;39(10):1651–6.

16. Zhou X, Otsuji Y, Yoshifuku S, et al. Impact of Atrial Fibrillation on Tricuspid and Mitral Annular Dilatation and Valvular Regurgitation. Circ J 2002;66(10): 913–6.

17. Kagiyama N, Hayashida A, Toki M, et al. Insufficient Leaflet Remodeling in Patients with Atrial Fibrillation: Association with the Severity of Mitral Regurgitation. Circ Cardiovasc Imaging 2017;10(3):e005451.

18. Kagiyama N, Mondillo S, Yoshida K, et al. Subtypes of Atrial Functional Mitral Regurgitation: Imaging Insights Into Their Mechanisms and Therapeutic Implications. JACC Cardiovasc Imaging 2020;13(3): 820–35.

19. Kim DH, Heo R, Handschumacher MD, et al. Mitral Valve Adaptation to Isolated Annular Dilation. Insights Into the Mechanism of Atrial Functional Mitral Regurgitation. JACC Cardiovasc Imaging 2017; 1–13. https://doi.org/10.1016/j.jcmg.2017.09.013.

20. Dal-Bianco JP, Aikawa E, Bischoff J, et al. Myocardial infarction alters adaptation of the tethered mitral valve. J Am Coll Cardiol 2016;67(3):275–87.

21. Grande-Allen KJ, Barber JE, Klatka KM, et al. Mitral valve stiffening in end-stage heart failure: Evidence of an organic contribution to functional mitral regurgitation. J Thorac Cardiovasc Surg 2005;130(3): 783–90.

22. Vandemaele P, Linden KV, Deferm S, et al. Alterations in Human Mitral Valve Mechanical Properties Secondary to Left Ventricular Remodeling : A Biaxial Mechanical Study. Front Cardiovasc Med 2022;9(June):1–16.

23. Bartko PE, Dal-Bianco JP, Guerrero JL, et al. Effect of Losartan on Mitral Valve Changes After Myocardial Infarction. J Am Coll Cardiol 2017;70(10): 1232–44.

24. Iborra-Egea O, Gálvez-Montón C, Roura S, et al. Mechanisms of action of sacubitril/valsartan on cardiac remodeling: a systems biology approach. Npj Syst Biol Appl 2017;3(1):1–8.

25. Tang Z, Fan YT, Wang Y, et al. Mitral Annular and Left Ventricular Dynamics in Atrial Functional Mitral Regurgitation: A Three-Dimensional and Speckle-Tracking Echocardiographic Study. J Am Soc Echocardiogr 2019;32(4):503–13.

26. Deferm S, Bertrand PB, Verhaert D, et al. Mitral Annular Dynamics in AF Versus Sinus Rhythm. JACC Cardiovasc Imaging 2022;15(1):1–13.

27. Silbiger JJ. Mechanistic insights into atrial functional mitral regurgitation: Far more complicated than just left atrial remodeling. Echocardiography 2019;36(1):164–9.

28. Bisbal F, Baranchuk A, Braunwald E, et al. Atrial Failure as a Clinical Entity: JACC Review Topic of the Week. J Am Coll Cardiol 2020;75(2):222–32.

29. Sanchis L, Gabrielli L, Andrea R, et al. Left atrial dysfunction relates to symptom onset in patients with heart failure and preserved left ventricular ejection fraction. Eur Heart J Cardiovasc Imaging 2015;16(1):62–7.

30. Reddy YNV, Obokata M, Verbrugge FH, et al. Atrial Dysfunction in Patients With Heart Failure With Preserved Ejection Fraction and Atrial Fibrillation. J Am Coll Cardiol 2020;76(9):1051–64.

31. Reddy YNV, Obokata M, Gersh BJ, et al. High Prevalence of Occult Heart Failure With Preserved Ejection Fraction Among Patients With Atrial Fibrillation and Dyspnea. Circulation 2018;137(5):534–5.

32. Patel RB, Shah SJ. Therapeutic Targeting of Left Atrial Myopathy in Atrial Fibrillation and Heart Failure with Preserved Ejection Fraction. JAMA Cardiol 2020;5(5):497–9.

33. Packer M, Lam CSP, Lund LH, et al. Interdependence of Atrial Fibrillation and Heart Failure with a Preserved Ejection Fraction Reflects a Common Underlying Atrial and Ventricular Myopathy. Circulation 2020; 4–6. https://doi.org/10.1161/CIRCULATIONAHA. 119.042996.

34. Tamargo M, Obokata M, Reddy YNV, et al. Functional mitral regurgitation and left atrial myopathy in heart failure with preserved ejection fraction. Eur J Heart Fail 2020;22(3):489–98.

35. Alkhouli M, Hahn RT, Petronio AS. Transcatheter Edge-to-Edge Repair for Atrial Functional Mitral Regurgitation. JACC Cardiovasc Interv 2022; 15(17):1741–7.

36. Simard T, Vemulapalli S, Jung RG, et al. Transcatheter Edge-to-Edge Repair in Patients with Severe Mitral Regurgitation and Cardiogenic Shock: TVT Registry Analysis. J Am Coll Cardiol 2022. https:// doi.org/10.1016/j.jacc.2022.09.006. S0735109722067675.

37. Chioncel O, Lainscak M, Seferovic PM, et al. Epidemiology and one-year outcomes in patients with chronic heart failure and preserved, mid-range and reduced ejection fraction: an analysis of the ESC Heart Failure Long-Term Registry Methods and results. Eur J Heart Fail 2017;19:1574–85.

38. Kajimoto K, Sato N, Takano T. Functional mitral regurgitation at discharge and outcomes in patients hospitalized for acute decompensated heart failure with a preserved or reduced ejection fraction. Eur J Heart Fail 2016;18(8):1051–9.

39. Lancellotti P, Tribouilloy C, Hagendorff A, et al. Recommendations for the echocardiographic assessment of native valvular regurgitation: An executive summary from the European Association of Cardiovascular Imaging. Eur Heart J Cardiovasc Imaging 2013;14(7):611–44.

40. Coisne A, Pontana F, Aghezzaf S, et al. Utility of Three-Dimensional Transesophageal Echocardiography for Mitral Annular Sizing in Transcatheter Mitral Valve Replacement Procedures: A Cardiac Computed Tomographic Comparative Study. J Am Soc Echocardiogr 2020;33(10):1245–52.e2.

41. Farhan S. Pathophysiology, Echocardiographic Diagnosis, and Treatment of Atrial Functional Mitral Regurgitation. J Am Coll Cardiol 2022; 80(24):17.

42. Gertz ZM, Herrmann HC, Lim DS, et al. Implications of Atrial Fibrillation on the Mechanisms of Mitral Regurgitation and Response to MitraClip in the COAPT Trial. Circ Cardiovasc Interv 2021;14: 424–32.

43. Zoghbi WA, Adams D, Bonow RO, et al. Recommendations for Noninvasive Evaluation of Native Valvular Regurgitation: A Report from the American Society of Echocardiography Developed in Collaboration with the Society for Cardiovascular Magnetic Resonance. J Am Soc Echocardiogr 2017; 30(4):303–71.

44. Hung J, Otsuji Y, Handschumacher MD, et al. Mechanism of dynamic regurgitant orifice area variation in functional mitral regurgitation. J Am Coll Cardiol 1999;33(2):538–45.

45. Marsan NA, Westenberg JJM, Ypenburg C, et al. Quantification of Functional Mitral Regurgitation by Real-Time 3D Echocardiography. Comparison With 3D Velocity-Encoded Cardiac Magnetic Resonance. JACC Cardiovasc Imaging 2009;2(11): 1245–52.

46. Zeng X, Levine RA, Hua L, et al. Diagnostic Value of Vena Contracta Area in the Quantification of Mitral Regurgitation Severity by Color Doppler 3D Echocardiography. Circ Cardiovasc Imaging 2011;4(5):506–13.

47. Kusunose K, Yamada H, Nishio S, et al. Index-beat assessment of left ventricular systolic and diastolic function during atrial fibrillation using myocardial strain and strain rate. J Am Soc Echocardiogr 2012;25(9):953–9.

48. Bartko PE, Arfsten H, Heitzinger G, et al. A Unifying Concept for the Quantitative Assessment of Secondary Mitral Regurgitation. J Am Coll Cardiol 2019;73(20):2506–17.

49. Grayburn PA, Sannino A, Packer M. Proportionate and Disproportionate Functional Mitral Regurgitation: A New Conceptual Framework That Reconciles the Results of the MITRA-FR and COAPT Trials. JACC Cardiovasc Imaging 2019;12(2): 353–62.

50. Packer M, Grayburn PA. New Evidence Supporting a Novel Conceptual Framework for Distinguishing Proportionate and Disproportionate Functional Mitral Regurgitation. JAMA Cardiol 2020;5(4): 469–75.

51. Mak GJ, Blanke P, Ong K, et al. Three-Dimensional Echocardiography Compared With Computed Tomography to Determine Mitral Annulus Size Before Transcatheter Mitral Valve Implantation. Circ Cardiovasc Imaging 2016;9(6):e004176.

52. Cawley PJ, Hamilton-Craig C, Owens DS, et al. Prospective Comparison of Valve Regurgitation Quantitation by Cardiac Magnetic Resonance

Imaging and Transthoracic Echocardiography. Circ Cardiovasc Imaging 2013;6(1):48–57.

53. Delgado V, Hundley WG. Added Value of Cardiovascular Magnetic Resonance in Primary Mitral Regurgitation. Circulation 2018;137(13):1361–3.

54. Marrouche NF, Wilber D, Hindricks G, et al. Association of Atrial Tissue Fibrosis Identified by Delayed Enhancement MRI and Atrial Fibrillation Catheter Ablation: The DECAAF Study. JAMA 2014;311(5):498–506.

55. Chelu MG, King JB, Kholmovski EG, et al. Atrial Fibrosis by Late Gadolinium Enhancement Magnetic Resonance Imaging and Catheter Ablation of Atrial Fibrillation: 5-Year Follow-Up Data. J Am Heart Assoc 2018;7(23):e006313.

56. Otto CM, Rick Nishimura CCA, Robert Bonow CCO, et al. 2020 ACC/AHA Guideline for the Management of Patients With Valvular Heart Disease. Circulation 2021;143. https://doi.org/10.1161/CIR.0000000000000923.

57. Vahanian A, Beyersdorf F, Praz F, et al. 2021 ESC/EACTS Guidelines for the management of valvular heart disease. Eur Heart J 2021;1–72. https://doi.org/10.1093/eurheartj/ehab395.

58. Reddy ST, Belden W, Doyle M, et al. Mitral regurgitation recovery and atrial reverse remodeling following pulmonary vein isolation procedure in patients with atrial fibrillation: A clinical observation proof-of-concept cardiac MRI study. J Interv Card Electrophysiol 2013;37(3):307–15.

59. Dell'Era G, Rondano E, Franchi E, et al. Atrial asynchrony and function before and after electrical cardioversion for persistent atrial fibrillation. Eur J Echocardiogr 2010;11(7):577–83.

60. Kirchhof P, Camm AJ, Goette A, et al. Early Rhythm-Control Therapy in Patients with Atrial Fibrillation. N Engl J Med 2020;1–11. https://doi.org/10.1056/NEJMoa2019422.

61. Masuda M, Sekiya K, Asai M, et al. Influence of catheter ablation for atrial fibrillation on atrial and ventricular functional mitral regurgitation. ESC Heart Fail 2022;9(3):1901–13.

62. Lam CSP, Voors AA, de Boer RA, et al. Heart failure with preserved ejection fraction: from mechanisms to therapies. Eur Heart J 2018;(June;1–13. https://doi.org/10.1093/eurheartj/ehy301.

63. Solomon SD, Vaduganathan M, Claggett B L, et al. Sacubitril/Valsartan across the Spectrum of Ejection Fraction in Heart Failure. Circulation 2020;352–61. https://doi.org/10.1161/CIRCULATIONAHA.119.044586.

64. Ducharme A, Swedberg K, Pfeffer MA, et al. Prevention of atrial fibrillation in patients with symptomatic chronic heart failure by candesartan in the Candesartan in Heart failure: Assessment of Reduction in Mortality and morbidity (CHARM) program. Am Heart J 2006;151(5):985–91.

65. Kang RT, Mitral F. Angiotensin Receptor Neprilysin Inhibitor for Functional Mitral Regurgitation : The PRIME Study. Circulation 2018. https://doi.org/10.1161/CIRCULATIONAHA.118.037077.

66. Januzzi JL, Omar AMS, Liu Y, et al. Association Between Sacubitril/Valsartan Initiation and Mitral Regurgitation Severity in Heart Failure With Reduced Ejection Fraction: The PROVE-HF Study. Circulation 2022;122:61693.

67. Solomon SD, McMurray JJV, Anand IS, et al. Angiotensin–neprilysin inhibition in heart failure with preserved ejection fraction. N Engl J Med 2019;381(17):1609–20.

68. John JV, McMurray MD, Milton Packer MD, et al. Angiotensin–Neprilysin Inhibition versus Enalapril in Heart Failure. N Engl J Med 2014. https://doi.org/10.1056/NEJMoa1409077.

69. Singh JSS, Burrell LM, Cherif M, et al. Sacubitril/valsartan: beyond natriuretic peptides. Heart 2017;103(20):1569–77.

70. Anker SD, Butler J, Filippatos G, et al. Empagliflozin in Heart Failure with a Preserved Ejection Fraction. N Engl J Med 2021;385(16):1451–61.

71. Solomon SD, McMurray JJV, Claggett B, et al. Dapagliflozin in Heart Failure with Mildly Reduced or Preserved Ejection Fraction. N Engl J Med 2022;387(12):1089–98.

72. Zelniker TA, Bonaca MP, Furtado RHM, et al. Effect of dapagliflozin on atrial fibrillation in patients with type 2 diabetes mellitus: Insights from the DECLARE-TIMI 58 Trial. Circulation 2020;1227–34.

73. Bax JJ, Braun J, Somer ST, et al. Restrictive annuloplasty and coronary revascularization in ischemic mitral regurgitation results in reverse left ventricular remodeling. Circulation 2004;110(11):103–9.

74. Bolling SF, Pagani FD, Deeb GM, et al. Intermediate-term outcome of mitral reconstruction in cardiomyopathy. J Thorac Cardiovasc Surg 1998;115(2):381–8.

75. Hung J, Papakostas L, Tahta SA, et al. Mechanism of recurrent ischemic mitral regurgitation after annuloplasty: Continued LV remodeling as a moving target. Circulation 2004;110(11):85–91.

76. Acker MA, Parides MK, Perrault LP, et al. Mitral-Valve Repair versus Replacement for Severe Ischemic Mitral Regurgitation. N Engl J Med 2014;370(1):23–32.

77. Goldstein D, Moskowitz AJ, Gelijns AC, et al. Two-Year Outcomes of Surgical Treatment of Severe Ischemic Mitral Regurgitation. N Engl J Med 2016;374(4):344–53.

78. Bertrand PB, Verbrugge FH, Verhaert D, et al. Mitral valve area during exercise after restrictive mitral valve annuloplasty: Importance of diastolic anterior leaflet tethering. J Am Coll Cardiol 2015;65(5):452–61.

79. Kubota K, Otsuji Y, Ueno T, et al. Functional mitral stenosis after surgical annuloplasty for ischemic

mitral regurgitation: Importance of subvalvular tethering in the mechanism and dynamic deterioration during exertion. J Thorac Cardiovasc Surg 2010; 140(3):617–23.

80. Wu AH, Aaronson KD, Bolling SF, et al. Impact of mitral valve annuloplasty on mortality risk in patients with mitral regurgitation and left ventricular systolic dysfunction. J Am Coll Cardiol 2005;45(3):381–7.

81. Smith PK, Puskas JD, Ascheim DD, et al. Surgical treatment of ischemic mitral valve regurgitation. NEJM 2005;11(4):228–31.

82. Michler RE, Smith PK, Parides MK, et al. Two-Year Outcomes of Surgical Treatment of Moderate Ischemic Mitral Regurgitation. N Engl J Med 2016;374(20):1932–41.

83. Deferm S, Bertrand PB, Verhaert D, et al. Outcome and durability of mitral valve annuloplasty in atrial secondary mitral regurgitation. Heart 2021;107(18): 1503–9.

84. Hirji SA, Cote CL, Javadikasgari H, et al. Atrial functional versus ventricular functional mitral regurgitation: Prognostic implications. J Thorac Cardiovasc Surg 2021. https://doi.org/10.1016/j.jtcvs.2020.12.098.

85. Takahashi Y, Shibata T, Hattori K, et al. Extended posterior leaflet extension for mitral regurgitation in giant left atrium. J Heart Valve Dis 2014;23(1): 88–90.

86. Yoon SH, Makar M, Kar S, et al. Outcomes After Transcatheter Edge-to-Edge Mitral Valve Repair According to Mitral Regurgitation Etiology and Cardiac Remodeling. JACC Cardiovasc Interv 2022; 15(17):1711–22.

87. Sodhi N, Asch FM, Ruf T, et al. Clinical Outcomes With Transcatheter Edge-to-Edge Repair in Atrial Functional MR From the EXPAND Study. JACC Cardiovasc Interv 2022;15(17):1723–30.

88. Tanaka T, Sugiura A, Öztürk C, et al. Transcatheter Edge-to-Edge Repair for Atrial Secondary Mitral Regurgitation. JACC Cardiovasc Interv 2022; 15(17):1731–40.

89. Doldi P, Stolz L, Orban M, et al. Transcatheter Mitral Valve Repair in Patients With Atrial Functional Mitral Regurgitation. JACC Cardiovasc Imaging 2022; 15(11):1843–51.

90. Schmidt FP, Von Bardeleben RS, Nikolai P, et al. Immediate effect of the MitraClip® procedure on mitral ring geometry in primary and secondary mitral regurgitation. Eur Heart J Cardiovasc Imaging 2013;14(9):851–7.

91. Kreidel F, Zaid S, Tamm AR, et al. Impact of Mitral Annular Dilation on Edge-to-Edge Therapy With MitraClip-XTR. Circ Cardiovasc Interv 2021;14(8): e010447.

92. Bax JJ, van der Bijl P. Etiology and Outcomes of Isolated Tricuspid Regurgitation. JACC Cardiovasc Imaging 2022;15(5):745–6.

93. Prihadi EA, Delgado V, Leon MB, et al. Morphologic Types of Tricuspid Regurgitation: Characteristics and Prognostic Implications. JACC Cardiovasc Imaging 2019;12(3):491–9.

94. Nemoto N, Lesser JR, Pedersen WR, et al. Pathogenic structural heart changes in early tricuspid regurgitation. J Thorac Cardiovasc Surg C 2015; 150(2):323. https://doi.org/10.1016/j.jtcvs.2015.05.009.

95. Utsunomiya H, Itabashi Y, Mihara H, et al. Functional Tricuspid Regurgitation Caused by Chronic Atrial Fibrillation: A Real-Time 3-Dimensional Transesophageal Echocardiography Study. Circ Cardiovasc Imaging 2017;10(1):e004897.

96. Utsunomiya H, Harada Y, Susawa H, et al. Tricuspid valve geometry and right heart remodelling: Insights into themechanismof atrial functional tricuspid regurgitation. Eur Heart J Cardiovasc Imaging 2020;21(10):1068–78.

97. Yamasaki N, Kondo F, Kubo T, et al. Severe Tricuspid Regurgitation in the Aged: Atrial Remodeling Associated With Long-Standing Atrial Fibrillation. J Cardiol 2006;48(6):315–23.

98. Muraru D, Caravita S, Guta AC. Functional Tricuspid Regurgitation and Atrial Fibrillation : Which Comes First , the Chicken or the Egg. Cardiovasc Imaging Case Rep 2020. https://doi.org/10.1016/j.case.2020.04.011.

99. Topilsky Y, Maltais S, Medina Inojosa J, et al. Burden of Tricuspid Regurgitation in Patients Diagnosed in the Community Setting. JACC Cardiovasc Imaging 2019;12(3):433–42.

100. Fender EA, Zack CJ, Nishimura RA. Isolated tricuspid regurgitation: Outcomes and therapeutic interventions. Heart 2018;104(10):798–806.

101. Topilsky Y, Nkomo VT, Vatury O, et al. Clinical outcome of isolated tricuspid regurgitation. JACC Cardiovasc Imaging 2014;7(12):1185–94.

102. Wang TKM, Akyuz K, Mentias A, et al. Contemporary Etiologies, Outcomes, and Novel Risk Score for Isolated Tricuspid Regurgitation. JACC Cardiovasc Imaging 2022;15(5):731–44.

103. Nath J, Foster E, Heidenreich PA. Impact of tricuspid regurgitation on long-term survival. J Am Coll Cardiol 2004;43(3):405–9.

104. Prihadi EA, van der Bijl P, Gursoy E, et al. Development of significant tricuspid regurgitation over time and prognostic implications: new insights into natural history. Eur Heart J 2018;39(39):3574–81.

105. Patlolla SH, Schaff HV, Nishimura RA, et al. Incidence and Burden of Tricuspid Regurgitation in Patients With Atrial Fibrillation. J Am Coll Cardiol 2022;80(24):2289–98.

106. Topilsky Y, Khanna A, Le Tourneau T, et al. Clinical context and mechanism of functional tricuspid regurgitation in patients with and without pulmonary hypertension. Circ Cardiovasc Imaging 2012;5(3):314–23.

107. Muraru D, Guta AC, Ochoa-Jimenez RC, et al. Functional Regurgitation of Atrioventricular Valves and Atrial Fibrillation: An Elusive Pathophysiological Link Deserving Further Attention. J Am Soc Echocardiogr 2020;33(1):42–53.

108. Silbiger JJ. Atrial functional tricuspid regurgitation: An underappreciated cause of secondary tricuspid regurgitation. Echocardiography 2019;36(5):954–7.

109. Hahn RT, Thomas JD, Khalique OK, et al. Imaging Assessment of Tricuspid Regurgitation Severity. JACC Cardiovasc Imaging 2019;12(3):469–90.

110. Badano LP, Hahn R, Zanella H, et al. Morphological Assessment of the Tricuspid Apparatus and Grading Regurgitation Severity in Patients With Functional Tricuspid Regurgitation: Thinking Outside the Box. JACC Cardiovasc Imaging 2019;12(4):652–64.

111. Hahn RT, Zamorano JL. The need for a new tricuspid regurgitation grading scheme. Eur Heart J Cardiovasc Imaging 2017;18(12):1342–3.

112. Hahn RT, Weckbach LT, Noack T, et al. Proposal for a Standard Echocardiographic Tricuspid Valve Nomenclature. JACC Cardiovasc Imaging 2021; 14(7):1299–305.

113. Guazzi M, Dixon D, Labate V, et al. RV Contractile Function and its Coupling to Pulmonary Circulation in Heart Failure With Preserved Ejection Fraction: Stratification of Clinical Phenotypes and Outcomes. JACC Cardiovasc Imaging 2017;10(10 Pt B): 1211–21.

114. Lorenz CH, Walker ES, Morgan VL, et al. Normal human right and left ventricular mass, systolic function, and gender differences by cine magnetic resonance imaging. J Cardiovasc Magn Reson 1999;1(1):7–21.

115. Sugeng L, Mor-Avi V, Weinert L, et al. Multimodality Comparison of Quantitative Volumetric Analysis of the Right Ventricle. JACC Cardiovasc Imaging 2010;3(1):10–8.

116. Asmarats L, Puri R, Latib A, et al. Transcatheter Tricuspid Valve Interventions: Landscape, Challenges, and Future Directions. J Am Coll Cardiol 2018;71(25):2935–56.

117. Agricola E, Asmarats L, Maisano F, et al. Imaging for Tricuspid Valve Repair and Replacement. JACC Cardiovasc Imaging 2021;14(1):61–111.

118. Soulat-Dufour L, Lang S, Addetia K, et al. Restoring Sinus Rhythm Reverses Cardiac Remodeling and Reduces Valvular Regurgitation in Patients With Atrial Fibrillation. J Am Coll Cardiol 2022;79(10): 951–61.

119. Vassileva CM, Shabosky J, Boley T, et al. Tricuspid valve surgery: The past 10 years from the Nationwide Inpatient Sample (NIS) database. J Thorac Cardiovasc Surg 2012;143(5):1043–9.

120. Zack CJ, Fender EA, Chandrashekar P, et al. National Trends and Outcomes in Isolated Tricuspid Valve Surgery. JACC J Am Coll Cardiol 2017.

121. Dreyfus J, Flagiello M, Bazire B, et al. Isolated tricuspid valve surgery: impact of aetiology and clinical presentation on outcomes. Eur Heart J 2020;41(45):4304–17.

122. Kundi H, Popma JJ, Cohen DJ, et al. Prevalence and Outcomes of Isolated Tricuspid Valve Surgery Among Medicare Beneficiaries. Am J Cardiol 2019; 123(1):132–8.

123. Ejiofor JI, Neely RC, Yammine M, et al. Surgical outcomes of isolated tricuspid valve procedures: repair versus replacement. Ann Cardiothorac Surg 2017;6(3):214–22.

124. Axtell AL, Bhambhani V, Moonsamy P, et al. Surgery Does Not Improve Survival in Patients With Isolated Severe Tricuspid Regurgitation. J Am Coll Cardiol 2019;74(6):715–25.

125. Patlolla SH, Schaff HV, Greason KL, et al. Early Right Ventricular Reverse Remodeling Predicts Survival After Isolated Tricuspid Valve Surgery. Ann Thorac Surg 2021;112(5):1402–9.

126. Lurz P, Stephan von Bardeleben R, Weber M, et al. Transcatheter Edge-to-Edge Repair for Treatment of Tricuspid Regurgitation. J Am Coll Cardiol 2021;77(3):229–39.

127. Kodali S, Hahn RT, Eleid MF, et al. Feasibility Study of the Transcatheter Valve Repair System for Severe Tricuspid Regurgitation. J Am Coll Cardiol 2021;77(4):345–56.

128. Donal E, Leurent G, Iung B. Are We Right to Believe in the Value of Transcatheter Treatment of Secondary Tricuspid Regurgitation? J Am Coll Cardiol 2021;77(3):240–2.

129. Ruf TF, Hahn RT, Kreidel F, et al. Short-Term Clinical Outcomes of Transcatheter Tricuspid Valve Repair With the Third-Generation MitraClip XTR System. JACC Cardiovasc Interv 2021;14(11):1231–40.

130. Praz F, Muraru D, Kreidel F, et al. Transcatheter treatment for tricuspid valve disease. EuroIntervention 2021;17(10):791–808.

Racial, Ethnic, and Gender Disparities in Valvular Heart Failure Management

Onyedika Ilonze, MD, MPH[a], Kendall Free, BS[b], Alexander Shinnerl, BA[c], Sabra Lewsey, MD, MPH[d], Khadijah Breathett, MD, MS[a],*

KEYWORDS

- Valvular heart disease • Heart failure • Mitral regurgitation • Aortic stenosis • Disparities
- Social determinants of health • Women's health • Racial disparities

KEY POINTS

- Valvular heart diseases are common as a cause or consequence of heart failure.
- Racial, ethnic, and gender disparities are present in medical and procedural management of valvular heart diseases.
- Implementation of strategies may reduce racial, ethnic, and gender disparities. Strategies should include universal health coverage, expanded access to subspecialist care, routine screening, increased enrollment in clinical trials, antiracist evaluation of institutional policies, and enhanced physician-patient relationship.

INTRODUCTION

Valvular heart disease (VHD) existing by itself or as a cause or consequence of heart failure (HF) is present in all populations, but disparities in treatments and outcomes exist depending on race, gender, and severity and type of valvular disease. Mitral regurgitation (MR), mitral stenosis (MS), aortic stenosis (AS), aortic regurgitation (AR), tricuspid regurgitation (TR), and rarely pulmonary valve disorders are commonly seen VHD in association with HF.

Racial and gender VHD disparities include differences in VHD risk, treatment, and outcomes. Disparities in VHD vary depending on severity and type of VHD. Black patients have an earlier age of onset and higher prevalence and age-adjusted mortality for HF when compared with other populations.[1] Women have worse outcomes from VHD such as mitral valve prolapse (MVP), and pregnant women with left-sided valvular disease such as MS and AS experience increased maternal morbidity and adverse fetal outcomes.[2,3] Advances in medications, interventional procedures, or cardiac surgery can improve outcomes for patients with VHD related to HF.

This article describes the prevalence of VHD associated with HF and disparities in minoritized racial and ethnic groups and women. The purpose is to better understand the mechanisms and etiologies of these disparities. Furthermore, this article proposes strategies to address racial, ethnic, and gender VHD disparities and improve health outcomes. By addressing these disparities and implementing solutions, health outcomes for all patients with VHD-associated HF may improve.

[a] Division of Cardiovascular Medicine, Krannert Cardiovascular Research Center, Indiana University, 1800 North Capitol Avenue, Indianapolis, IN 46202, USA; [b] Department of Biofunction Research, Tokyo Medical and Dental University, 2 Chome-3-10 Kanda Surugadai, Chiyoda City, Tokyo 101-0062, Japan; [c] College of Medicine, Indiana University, 340 West 10th Street, Indianapolis, IN 46202, USA; [d] Division of Cardiology, Department of Medicine, Johns Hopkins University School of Medicine, 601 North Caroline Street, 7th Floor, Baltimore, MD 21287, USA
* Corresponding author.
E-mail address: kbreath@iu.edu

Heart Failure Clin 19 (2023) 379–390
https://doi.org/10.1016/j.hfc.2023.02.009
1551-7136/23/© 2023 Elsevier Inc. All rights reserved.

DISPARITIES IN MITRAL VALVE DISEASES ASSOCIATED WITH HEART FAILURE
Epidemiology of Mitral Regurgitation, Mitral Valve Prolapse, and Mitral Stenosis

Mitral regurgitation (MR) is a common valvular disease that can be classified as primary or secondary. MR has an estimated prevalence of approximately 1.7%, which increases to approximately 9.3% in those greater than 75 years of age.[4] Primary MR is caused by a structural abnormality of the mitral valve (MV), usually caused by rheumatic heart disease in under-resourced countries or by degenerative valve disease, predominantly mitral valve prolapse (MVP) in the United States.[5] Secondary MR is caused by left ventricular dysfunction and/or dilatation with associated electrical/mechanical abnormalities and absence of organic valvular disease and is more common than primary MR. Secondary MR is a predictor of poor clinical outcomes in patients with HF with reduced left ventricular ejection fraction (HFrEF) and associated with a threefold risk of HF and a twofold risk of death compared to patients without MR.[6,7] The severity of secondary MR is associated with the risk of HF and all-cause mortality.[8] In a retrospective study of patients with dilated cardiomyopathy, 24% of patients had quantitatively assessed severe secondary MR, which was a predictor of death and HF hospitalizations at 2.5 years of follow-up.[8]

MVP and MR impacts patients differentially by sex and by race. MVP is a valvular disease characterized by excessive MV leaflet displacement into the left atrium in systole usually caused by myxomatous degeneration. The prognosis of MVP is usually benign, but serious sequelae can occur, most frequently resulting in severe MR.[9] It is more common in women. A large health system in the United Kingdom showed that Black patients had a higher prevalence of secondary MR caused by restricted leaflets than White or Asian patients, likely because of higher prevalence of nonischemic cardiomyopathy.[10] Black women have more cardiovascular risk factors and higher risk of HF and death before HF and thus represent a more vulnerable population when concomitant MR or MVP is present.[11]

MS presentation and treatment vary from MR. MS is usually caused by rheumatic heart disease and is common in under-resourced countries and in US immigrant populations.[5] It is characterized by leaflet thickening (or calcification), nodularity, and commissural fusion, all of which result in MV. Efficacy of medical treatment by drugs for severe MS is poor, and interventional treatment is preferred except in cases of a strong contraindication.

Disparities in treatments and outcome of mitral regurgitation, mitral valve prolapse and mitral stenosis

Gender and racial differences exist regarding MV pathology, operative strategy, and long-term outcomes. Women have a higher prevalence of MV calcification, rheumatic MV disease, and increased leaflet thickening, which can be challenging for MV repair.[12,13] Compared with men, women are less likely to undergo MV repair, but when they do receive treatment, they have more advanced disease stages, and consequently higher operative mortality and reduced long-term survival.[14] Women with MVP are less likely to undergo cardiac valve surgery than men and have higher rates of survival for mild MR, yet experience worse survival rates for severe MR associated with MVP.[13] Women also experience higher risk for morbidity and mortality when undergoing combined valve and bypass surgery. Among patients with MVP and severe MR, women with severe disease have worse survival and lower surgery rates than men.[3,13] Women with MR are more likely to undergo prosthetic MV replacement, have concomitant tricuspid valve surgery, and have worse postoperative long-term survival.[3] It is unclear how much of these findings are caused by late diagnoses or delayed referral. Clinician bias is a known factor contributing to lack of referral or discriminatory decision-making for other cardiovascular disease diseases.[15–17]

Racial differences exist in the prescription of guideline-directed medical therapy (GDMT), which remains first-line therapy for secondary MR and HFrEF.[18,19] A national community surveillance of hospitalized HF events in the United States demonstrated that optimal GDMT was prescribed in about 10% of patients at hospital discharge.[20] This underprescription of GDMT may disproportionately worsen clinical outcomes of secondary MR in Black patients who have higher rates of nonischemic cardiomyopathy.[10]

Cardiac resynchronization therapy (CRT) is not optimally used across populations. CRT with optimal GDMT is the next therapeutic option for eligible patients with secondary MR and HFrEF and should be performed before MV procedural interventions. It is recommended in patients with HFrEF and left bundle branch block, in sinus rhythm with New York Heart Association functional class II to IV symptoms on GDMT with left ventricular (LV) ejection fraction of no more than 35%.[21] CRT reduces leaflet tethering and closing forces on the MV, improves leaflet coaptation thereby restoring synchronous LV contraction, decreases LV size, improves LV systolic function, and reduces secondary MR over 3 to 6 months of follow-up.[6,22] Black patients are less likely than White patients to receive implantable cardioverter defibrillators after adjusting for demographics, clinical characteristics, and socioeconomic factors.[23] An examination of a national registry found that Black and Hispanic patients who were eligible for CRT with defibrillator were less likely to receive therapy compared with White patients.[24] These disparities in CRT utilization have persisted over time, with underuse of CRT in Black patients and women.[25] The Affordable Care Act (ACA) was associated with increased CRT access for White but not Black or Hispanic populations.[26]

Data regarding use of transcatheter edge-to-edge mitral valve repair (TMVR) are limited by race. The TMVR MitraClip (Abbott, Abbott Park, Illinois) is the most widely adopted device and has been studied in 2 randomized, controlled trials among patients with HFrEF and secondary MR.[27,28] The racial composition of the participants was not reported in these trials. A propensity score matched outcomes analysis from 2012 to 2016 showed that only 8.6% of TMVR procedures were performed in Black patients with an unchanged proportion of Black patients over time despite increase in procedural volume.[29] Black patients undergoing TMVR were more likely to be younger and female compared with White patients.[29] White patients had higher in-hospital cardiac arrest and pacemaker insertion and shorter median length of stay when compared with Black patients.[29] Another study showed no gender differences in rates of TMVR and no difference in in-hospital mortality and major complications for TMVR among women compared with men.[30]

MV repair is preferred over MV replacement as the treatment of primary MR but is allocated disparately by race. MV repair is ideal because of lower operative/long-term mortality, improved preservation of LV function, avoidance of anticoagulation, decreased risk of thromboembolic complications, endocarditis, and long-term freedom from reoperation.[31] A retrospective analysis found that patients undergoing MV surgery were younger (45.6 ± 14.4 versus 60.5 ± 15.3 years), less likely to undergo MV repair, and had higher incidence of comorbidities, whereas White patients (n = 1,302, 91.4%) underwent repair more commonly with degenerative MV disease.[32] No differences were found in the incidence of postoperative complications or hospital mortality (2.4% Black race versus 5.1% White race, p=.19).[32] An administrative database analysis found that Black and Hispanic patients had a more emergent presentation for MV surgery, underwent MV repair less often, were more likely to have MV replacement, and had a higher length

of stay when compared with White patients.[33] A 10-year analysis of care in Michigan demonstrated higher likelihood of MV repair for White patients than other racial groups (White 66%, Black 53.3%, other race 57%; P<.001) and similar operative mortality across racial groups (White 3.7%, Black 4.6%, other 4.5%; P=.36).[34]

MS treatments vary by country wealth. Negative chronotropic agents and diuretics are the mainstay for medical therapy control of heart rate in symptomatic MS. Correction of secondary conditions such as anemia, fever, infection, and volume overload can also be beneficial. Surgical options include closed or open valvotomy and MV replacement. Closed valvotomy is mostly done in under-resourced countries, while percutaneous balloon valvuloplasty allows controlled reconstruction of the valves, and simultaneous tricuspid valve repair or MV replacement to be performed if indicated.

DISPARITIES IN AORTIC VALVE DISEASE
Epidemiology of Aortic Stenosis and Aortic Regurgitation

Aortic stenosis (AS) is a common valvular heart disease and mainly a disease of aging.[35] The most common cause of AS in the United States is calcific AV disease, but rheumatic heart disease is often a cause in US immigrant populations, under-resourced countries, and in patients with congenital bicuspid valve. A meta-analysis of older subjects 75 years of age or older in Europe and North America demonstrated a population prevalence of AS of 12.4% and a prevalence of severe AS of 3.4%.[36] Aortic regurgitation (AR) is the diastolic reversal of blood flow from the aorta into the left ventricle. In the Framingham study, the prevalence of AR was estimated as 4.9%, and moderate and severe AR occurred in 0.5% of the study population; AR was observed in 13% of men and 8.5% of women.[37] The incidence and severity of AR increase with age, peaking at 40 to 60 years.[37]

Black patients may have lower prevalence of AS than White patients.[38,39] Studies have demonstrated a lower prevalence of AS in Black patients and other under-represented ethnic groups.[40–42] The aortic stenosis paradox is a phenomenon whereby under-represented racial and ethnic groups have more cardiovascular risk factors relative to White patients but have a lower burden of AS.[39–41] However, it is unclear how much of this related to improper diagnoses. A single-center study of 272,429 patients with retrospective echocardiographic data observed severe AS in 0.29% of Black and 0.91% of White patients, and Black patients were less likely to present with either degenerative AS or bicuspid AV disease.[38] It remains unclear if this is related to underdiagnosis or less AS in Black patients. The best assessment of valvular disease prevalence would require standardized echocardiogram for all population groups irrespective of symptoms and clinical examination to determine the prevalence of disease.

Disparities in Treatments and Outcomes of Aortic Stenosis

Traditionally, surgical aortic valve replacement (SAVR), which improves symptoms and survival, was the mainstay of intervention. Transcatheter aortic-valve replacement (TAVR) has been shown to be effective in patients with low-, intermediate-, and high-risk AS with favorable long-term outcomes.[43–46] TAVR is the preferred option for AS in certain subsets of patients (advanced age, poor LV function, or coexisting disorders) at increased risk for operative complications or death.

Black patients are poorly represented in published series of surgical aortic valve replacement and clinical trials of TAVR. The magnitude of under-representation in clinical trials is staggering, as only 2.7% in the high-risk pool (19 out of 699) were Black patients in the TAVR PARTNER trial.[46] There are currently no data on the literature on equity in access or utilization of aortic regurgitation interventions or surgery among women and Black and Indigenous People of Color (BIPOC).

Disparities in Structural Cardiology Referrals

Black patients with severe AS are less likely to be referred for structural interventions. A single-center study showed that Black patients with severe AS were less likely to be referred to cardiology, more likely to decline an intervention, or be lost to follow-up.[47] For every $10,000 increase in income, the odds of receiving TAVR increased by 10% ($p=.05$), suggesting that income significantly influenced the odds of receiving TAVR.[47]

Racial and gender disparities in referral for cardiovascular treatment may be extrapolated to TAVR. Cardiology referrals and follow-up appointments have been less likely to be made for Hispanic and Black HF patients and patients with lower socioeconomic position compared with White patients and patients with higher socioeconomic position.[48] A national study revealed that Black patients were less likely to receive care by a cardiologist than White patients when presenting with primary diagnosis of HF requiring intensive care.[49] Physician racial bias has been identified as a possible contributing factor for unequitable referrals.[49]

Disparities in Treatments and Outcomes of Aortic Stenosis

Racial disparities exist in referral patterns for SAVR. A retrospective single-center cohort design of 952 patients (423 White, 376 Black, and 153 Hispanic) found that after adjusting for clinical and echocardiographic variables, Black patients were younger and more likely to have Medicaid as payer, had more advanced kidney disease, and were less likely to be referred to cardiac surgery for treatment of AV disease when compared with White patients.[50] Overall SAVR rates increased, but women and Black patients had lower rates of SAVR and higher mortality than men and White patients in a large cross-sectional cohort study of Medicare fee-for-service beneficiaries between 1999 and 2011.[51]

Hospitalization for AS varies by racial and ethnicity.[52] Hospitalization with AS is less common in Black and Hispanic patients than in White patients.[52] In hospitalized patients with AS, Black race is associated with a lower incidence of both SAVR and TAVR compared with White patients, whereas Hispanic patients have a similar incidence of both.[52,53] Black patients with severe AS may suffer greater morbidity and mortality compared with other racial and ethnic groups.[54]

Under-represented racial/ethnic groups have lower rates of TAVR, and data are mixed on some of the outcomes. A review of a national registry found under-representation of minoritized racial groups among patients undergoing TAVR in the United States. Of the 70,221 patients who underwent TAVR, 91.3%, 3.8%, 3.4%, and 1.5% were White, Black, Hispanic, and Asian/American Indian/Pacific Islander race respectively.[55] No differences of in-hospital mortality, myocardial infarction, stroke, major bleeding, vascular complications, or new pacemaker requirements were observed, but Black and Hispanic patients had more HF hospitalizations when compared with White patients.[55]

Structural heart interventions were performed less frequently in Black and Hispanic patients compared with White patients in a retrospective national inpatient study of 106,119 weighted hospitalizations for TAVR, TMVR, and left atrial appendage occlusion.[56] Utilization rates were higher in White patients compared with Black and Hispanic patients for TAVR (43.1 versus 18.0 versus 21.1), TMVR (5.0 versus 3.2 versus 3.2), and left atrial appendage occlusion (6.6 versus 2.1 versus 3.5), respectively ($P<.001$). No differences in the adjusted in-hospital mortality or key complications between patients of all races following TAVR, TMVR, or left atrial appendage occlusion were observed. Hispanic patients had modestly higher cost with TMVR and left atrial appendage occlusion when compared with White patients.[56]

Black patients are less frequently referred for cardiac catheterization, percutaneous coronary interventions, and coronary artery bypass graft surgery than White patients.[57,58] These differences cannot be accounted for on the basis of health insurance or socioeconomic status.[59] As the population of VHD candidates and treatment options for valvular diseases expand, ensuring equity in referrals and interventions towards all groups is important to improve outcomes.

Disparities in Tricuspid Valve Disease

Epidemiology of tricuspid regurgitation
Tricuspid regurgitation (TR) affects 1.6 million US adults and is increasingly recognized for its increased associated mortality, regardless of pulmonary artery pressures or LV function.[60,61] TR impacts a higher percentage of women than men, and the Framingham study suggested TR of mild or more severity is seen in 14.8% of men and 18.4% of women and is strongly associated with age.[37,62,63] Population cohort estimates of TR have varied.[62,64] Observed mortality associated with TR is closely linked to TR severity and speed of development.[60] Functional TR, marked by tricuspid annular dilation and adverse right ventricular (RV) remodeling, is most commonly observed in the setting of left heart disease, right ventricular dysfunction, and pulmonary hypertension.[62] Primary TR is less common than secondary TR, and is due to intrinsic structural abnormalities in the valve or sub valvular aparatus.[65] It may result from infective endocarditis, with intracardiac device placement, rheumatic heart disease, carcinoid syndrome, or congenital malformations (ie, Ebstein's anomaly).[66]

Disparities in tricuspid valve interventions
Decisions for intervention for TR should be taken in the context of TR severity, associated RV remodeling, and comorbid conditions.[67] Isolated tricuspid valve (TV) repair and replacement bear high in-hospital mortality risk (8.8 to 10.9%), high risk of pacemaker implantation, and significant risk of new dialysis.[68] Thus, most TV surgery is performed concomitant to other cardiac surgery, and few isolated TV surgeries are performed. A retrospective analysis of isolated TV surgery did not show significant sex-based differences in 30-day mortality, 5-year survival, or 5-year freedom from TV reoperation.[69] Transcatheter tricuspid valve repair (TTVR) is an emerging option for intervention, with and without a concomitant TMVR

and is in active trial development, and its role in clinical practice is still being defined.[70,71] Rehospitalization for HF is common in the first 30 days after TTVR; however, 1-year outcomes suggest reduction in HF hospitalization and death, improvement in New York Heart Association functional class, and improved self-assessed health status in patients with procedural success.[71,72]

Trial inclusion for tricuspid valve intervention varies by sex and patient race and ethnicity. Women have been well-represented in transcatheter tricuspid intervention trials, comprising more than 60% of some cohorts given increased prevalence of TR in women; however, little to no trial representation has been reported for BIPOC.[70,72] Effectively, no data regarding equity of access to or utilization of transcatheter tricuspid interventions in women and BIPOC have been published to date.

Disparities in pulmonic valve disease
Pulmonic stenosis is common in the setting of congenital heart disease.[73] Pulmonary regurgitation (PR) is observed in 5% of structurally normal hearts,[74] but more commonly is seen following surgical or balloon valvuloplasty intervention for RV outflow tract obstruction, particularly in the case of Tetralogy of Fallot.[73] Surgical and transcatheter pulmonic valve replacement are both interventions for pulmonary regurgitation in appropriately selected patients.

There are no current data on the literature on equity in access or utilization of pulmonary valve interventions among women and BIPOC. Pulmonary valve repair timing has focused on development of RV dilation, HF, and arrhythmias in hopes of circumventing sudden cardiac death. Sex-based differences in volumetric assessments by cardiac MRI may further inform optimal timing for pulmonary valve repair following Tetralogy of Fallot repair. Gaps in transition from the pediatric cardiology to the adult congenital heart disease specialist have been implicated as factors in losing patients with congenital heart disease, with some being lost to follow up.[75]

STRATEGIES FOR BRIDGING DISPARITIES IN THERAPIES FOR TREATMENT OF VALVULAR HEART DISEASES IN HEART FAILURE

Women, patients who identify as BIPOC, and individuals with lower socioeconomic position have worse HF outcomes and poorer access to and utilization of valvular interventions. These disparate outcomes warrant focused attention to devise and employ effective solutions to bridge disparities in outcomes and therapeutic utilization in VHD and HF (**Table 1, Fig. 1**).

Table 1
Disparities and strategies in selected valvular heart diseases associated with heart failure

Therapeutics for Valvular Heart Disease Associated with Heart Failure	Disparities in Women and BIPOC	Strategies to Address Disparities
Mitral regurgitation • GDMT • CRT • TMVR • MVR MS • Balloon valvuloplasty • Heart rate control AS • TAVR • SAVR Tricuspid regurgitation • GDMT • TTVR Pulmonary regurgitation/ stenosis in CHD • Pulmonary valve repair	• Inadequate GDMT prescription • Lower CRT implants • Lower TMVR procedures • Less MVR and worse MVR outcomes in women • Under-resourced communities and immigrants • Untreated rheumatic heart disease • Underdiagnosis • Disparities in structural cardiology referrals • Under-representation in clinical trials • Underutilization of TAVR and SAVR • Paucity of randomized trials • Underdiagnosis • Delay in transition from pediatric cardiologist to ACHD cardiologist	• Address lack of insurance through universal health coverage • Address poor distribution of cardiologists through physician incentives and telemedicine • Automated valvular disease screening and structural cardiology referral • Larger BIPOC participation in trials and diversifying leadership of clinical trials • Addressing policies that contribute to systemic racism and bias and worsen SDOH; providing gender/race concordant clinician-patient relationships for mistreated populations • Transition to adult congenital heart disease specialists

Abbreviations: ACHD, adult congenital heart disease; BIPOC, Black and indigenous people of color; CHD, congenital heart disease; CRT, cardiac resynchronization therapy; GDMT, guideline-directed medical therapy; MVR, mitral valve repair; SAVR, surgical aortic valve replacement; SDOH, social determinants of health; TAVR, transcatheter aortic valve replacement; TMVR, transcatheter mitral valve repair; TTVR, transcatheter tricuspid valve repair.

Access to CV providers, interventions, and GDMT is fundamental to receiving appropriate, timely therapy for VHD and HF. Lack of insurance or underinsurance limits attainment of these essentials to care. The primary driver for inadequate insurance is cost of coverage. High out-of-pocket cost contributes to delays in care, and with regards to VHD, delayed presentations portend poor outcomes and limited interventional options. Systemic review of Medicaid expansion under the ACA suggests that insurance coverage increased among those eligible, particularly minoritized racial and ethnic groups.[76] Hispanic patients had a higher probability of receiving all GDMT if they were residents of early adopter rather than nonadopter states of the ACA Medicaid Expansion, irrespective of timing of the ACA.[77] Medicaid expansion has also been associated with increased access to heart transplantation in Black patients.[78] Expansion of coverage may be of particular benefit for younger patients with VHD and HF. Although Medicare has near universal coverage of those over age 65, with fewer than 1% not covered, affordable prescription coverage remains a challenge for many

older adults. Affordable health and prescription drug coverage may decrease disparities by improving access to HF services and therapies among minoritized racial and ethnic groups and those experiencing economic hardship.[79]

Risk calculators that predict postsurgical risk and hence decision to offer cardiac surgery can be fraught with bias. The Society of Thoracic Surgeons risk calculator is an online risk calculator that predicts the risk of adverse outcomes and mortality after cardiac surgery.[80] There should be reconsideration of the use of race in risk calculators since race is a social construct with no biologic basis. Understanding how social determinants of health and structural racism contribute to outcomes may be more useful. Additionally, bias towards Black patients may lead to less likelihood of recommending cardiac surgery, hence perpetuating inequity.

Incorporation of quality metrics surrounding indicated valvular interventions and standardization of valve referral consideration, as has been proposed with other HF therapies, may also bridge disparity gaps.[81] As there may be limited numbers

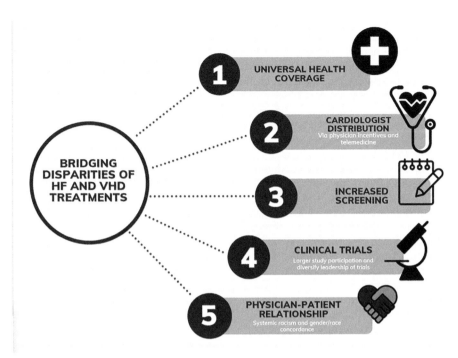

Fig. 1. Bridging disparities of heart failure and valvular heart disease treatments.

and geographic clustering of HF cardiologists, echocardiographers, and structural interventionalists, consideration should be given to novel care delivery models that leverage telemedicine and outreach clinics in which patients can remain local and still receive streamlined specialty cardiovascular care. Central to this consideration are mechanisms to increase community-based screening of VHD for patients with indications by history, symptoms, and examination, with increased awareness of the populations at highest risk.

Diverse clinical trial representation is an imperative for valvular intervention trials. Utilization of evidenced-based, life-saving valve interventions too often followed a path of diminished and delayed access to diverse and under-resourced communities. Black patients are decreasingly represented in HF therapeutic trials.[82] Women have historically been under-represented in HF clinical trials.[83,84] Policies supporting community-based trial design and enrollment and mandating transparency in the demographics of enrollees are needed. Making clinical trials more inclusive requires diversification of clinical trialist, their ancillary teams, and trial leadership with individuals who can authentically engage diverse communities.[85] Diverse trial leadership should be nurtured and trained in cultural competency and effective messaging to build trust with diverse communities.[86,87] Equitable representation of diverse communities must be demanded by the cardiovascular community, in pursuit of the best possible outcomes for all patients.[88]

VHD and HF therapies are particularly vulnerable to gatekeeper effects. That is, the interfacing clinical provider can advance or delay a patient's ability to access critical, guideline-directed therapies. This has been seen in referral practices for advanced HF therapeutics broadly.[89] Surgical or transcatheter valve repair or replacement candidacy is thus largely contingent upon provider referral. Bias has been observed in physician decision making regarding advanced HF candidacy; such studies have not commenced for VHD interventions.[90] The patient-physician partnership and communication may be influenced by several social factors.[91] Some studies suggest that race discordant dyads may be perceived as more difficult by providers.[92] Ethnic concordance in other studies has been shown to ease interaction and improve knowledge retention, even in patients reporting lower literacy.[93] Patient-physician communications may be of poor quality when clinicians hold unconscious bias, are unable to execute a shared-decision making skillset, or are lacking cultural competence.[94] Patients are particularly vulnerable to these poor-quality encounters when they have limited English proficiency, low health literacy, and are members of racial/ethnic minority groups.[94] Strategic interventions to address implicit bias among providers, shared-decision making, and cultural competency are imperative to improve patient-physician communication and deconstruct barriers to appropriate and timely referral for VHD and HF interventions. Ensuring seamless transition of adolescent and young patients with congenital heart disease from the pediatric cardiologist to the adult congenital heart disease cardiologist can improve health-related knowledge and self-management and reduce need for urgent valvular interventions.[95]

Cultural competency training must include education regarding the social and structural determinants of health (SDOH) and their impact on VHD and HF burden and outcomes. The SDOH are defined as the nonmedical factors that impact health and involve neighborhoods and housing, economic stability, health care access and delivery, education, and social context.[96] Fundamental to understanding the role of SDOH is recognizing structural racism and its primary contribution to adverse HF and VHD outcomes in BIPOC.[97] Equity-focused interventions must take a primary role in remodeling HF outcomes in diverse communities.[98]

SUMMARY

Disparities in the prevalence and treatment of HF and VHD persist for Black, Hispanic, American Indian, and female patients. Black patients experience the highest burden of HF. Women experience heightened burdens of VHD. Various factors contribute to the higher burden of HF and VHD in minoritized racial and ethnic groups and women that must be addressed by facing systemic racism and bias. Approaches necessary to reduce health disparities in HF and VHD should include considerations for universal health coverage, increased access to subspecialist care and screening, increased diverse trial participation, and antiracist evaluation of institutional policies.

CLINICS CARE POINTS

- When identifying symptomatic valvular disease, assess for appropriate pharmacological and nonpharmacological treatment. Be wary of risk prediction calculators that include race or ethnicity.
- Avoid delaying referrals to specialists. Specialists can provide multidisciplinary care.
- In the setting of severe valvular disease, assess how current institutional policies could worsen access to care for women and minoritized racial and ethnic groups. Develop institutional strategies to prevent disparities and reassess for need to change policies further.

FUNDING

This study was funded by Dr K. Breathett's research support from the National Heart, Lung, and Blood Institute, United States (NHLBI) K01HL142848, R56HL159216, R01HL159216, and L30HL148881.

REFERENCES

1. Rethy L, Petito LC, Vu THT, et al. Trends in the prevalence of self-reported heart failure by race/ethnicity and age from 2001 to 2016. JAMA Cardiology 2020; 5(12):1425–9.
2. Hameed A, Karaalp IS, Tummala PP, et al. The effect of valvular heart disease on maternal and fetal outcome of pregnancy. J Am Coll Cardiol 2001;37(3):893–9.
3. Seeburger J, Eifert S, Pfannmuller B, et al. Gender differences in mitral valve surgery. Thorac Cardiovasc Surg 2013;61(1):42–6.
4. Nkomo VT, Gardin JM, Skelton TN, et al. Burden of valvular heart diseases: a population-based study. Lancet (London, England) 2006;368(9540):1005–11.
5. Writing Committee M, Otto CM, Nishimura RA, et al. 2020 ACC/AHA guideline for the management of patients with valvular heart disease: a report of the American College of Cardiology/American Heart Association Joint Committee on Clinical Practice Guidelines. J Am Coll Cardiol 2021;77(4): e25–197.
6. Asgar AW, Mack MJ, Stone GW. Secondary mitral regurgitation in heart failure: pathophysiology, prognosis, and therapeutic considerations. J Am Coll Cardiol 2015;65(12):1231–48.
7. Trichon BH, Felker GM, Shaw LK, et al. Relation of frequency and severity of mitral regurgitation to survival among patients with left ventricular systolic dysfunction and heart failure. Am J Cardiol 2003; 91(5):538–43.
8. Rossi A, Dini FL, Faggiano P, et al. Independent prognostic value of functional mitral regurgitation in patients with heart failure. A quantitative analysis of 1256 patients with ischaemic and non-ischaemic dilated cardiomyopathy. Heart (British Cardiac Society) 2011;97(20):1675–80.
9. Hayek E, Gring CN, Griffin BP. Mitral valve prolapse. Lancet (London, England) 2005;365(9458):507–18.
10. Hayward C, Monteiro R, Ferreira A, et al. Racial differences in the aetiology of mitral valve disease. Eur Heart J Qual Care Clin Outcomes 2021;7(4): e3–4.
11. Breathett K, Leng I, Foraker RE, et al. Risk factor burden, heart failure, and survival in women of different ethnic groups: insights from the women's health initiative. Circulation Heart Failure 2018;11(5): e004642.
12. Mantovani F, Clavel MA, Michelena HI, et al. Comprehensive imaging in women with organic mitral

regurgitation: implications for clinical outcome. JACC Cardiovasc Imaging 2016;9(4):388–96.

13. Avierinos JF, Inamo J, Grigioni F, et al. Sex differences in morphology and outcomes of mitral valve prolapse. Ann Intern Med 2008;149(11):787–95.

14. Vassileva CM, McNeely C, Mishkel G, et al. Gender differences in long-term survival of Medicare beneficiaries undergoing mitral valve operations. Ann Thorac Surg 2013;96(4):1367–73.

15. Wenger NK. Women and coronary heart disease: a century after Herrick: understudied, underdiagnosed, and undertreated. Circulation 2012;126(5):604–11.

16. Daugherty SL, Blair IV, Havranek EP, et al. Implicit gender bias and the use of cardiovascular tests among cardiologists. J Am Heart Assoc 2017;6(12). https://doi.org/10.1161/JAHA.117.006872.

17. Breathett K, Yee E, Pool N, et al. Association of gender and race with allocation of advanced heart failure therapies. JAMA Netw Open 2020;3(7):e2011044.

18. Ilonze O, Free K, Breathett K. Unequitable heart failure therapy for black, hispanic and american-indian patients. Card Fail Rev 2022;8:e25.

19. Nayak A, Hicks AJ, Morris AA. Understanding the complexity of heart failure risk and treatment in black patients. Circulation Heart Failure 2020;13(8):e007264.

20. Mathews L, Ding N, Sang Y, et al. Racial differences in trends and prognosis of guideline-directed medical therapy for heart failure with reduced ejection fraction: the atherosclerosis risk in communities (ARIC) surveillance study. J Racial Ethn Health Disparities 2022. https://doi.org/10.1007/s40615-021-01202-5.

21. Heidenreich PA, Bozkurt B, Aguilar D, et al. 2022 AHA/ACC/HFSA guideline for the management of heart failure: a report of the American College of Cardiology/American Heart Association Joint Committee on Clinical Practice Guidelines. Circulation 2022;145(18):e895–1032.

22. Spartera M, Galderisi M, Mele D, et al. Role of cardiac dyssynchrony and resynchronization therapy in functional mitral regurgitation. European Heart Journal Cardiovascular Imaging 2016;17(5):471–80.

23. Thomas KL, Al-Khatib SM, Kelsey RC 2nd, et al. Racial disparity in the utilization of implantable-cardioverter defibrillators among patients with prior myocardial infarction and an ejection fraction of <or=35. Am J Cardiol 2007;100(6):924–9.

24. Farmer SA, Kirkpatrick JN, Heidenreich PA, et al. Ethnic and racial disparities in cardiac resynchronization therapy. Heart Rhythm 2009;6(3):325–31.

25. Sridhar AR, Yarlagadda V, Parasa S, et al. Cardiac resynchronization therapy: us trends and disparities in utilization and outcomes. Circ Arrhythm Electrophysiol 2016;9(3):e003108.

26. Mwansa H, Barry I, Knapp SM, et al. Association between the affordable care act medicaid expansion and receipt of cardiac resynchronization therapy by race and ethnicity. J Am Heart Assoc 2022;11(19):e026766.

27. Obadia JF, Messika-Zeitoun D, Leurent G, et al. Percutaneous repair or medical treatment for secondary mitral regurgitation. N Engl J Med 2018;379(24):2297–306.

28. Stone GW, Lindenfeld J, Abraham WT, et al. Transcatheter mitral-valve repair in patients with heart failure. N Engl J Med 2018;379(24):2307–18.

29. Elbadawi A, Mahmoud K, Elgendy IY, et al. Racial disparities in the utilization and outcomes of transcatheter mitral valve repair: insights from a national database. Cardiovasc Revascularization Med 2020;21(11):1425–30.

30. Elbadawi A, Elzeneini M, Thakker R, et al. Sex differences in in-hospital outcomes of transcatheter mitral valve repair (from a national database). Am J Cardiol 2020;125(9):1391–7.

31. Gillinov AM, Blackstone EH, Nowicki ER, et al. Valve repair versus valve replacement for degenerative mitral valve disease. J Thorac Cardiovasc Surg 2008;135(4):885–93, 893 e1-e893.

32. DiGiorgi PL, Baumann FG, O'Leary AM, et al. Mitral valve disease presentation and surgical outcome in African-American patients compared with white patients. Ann Thorac Surg 2008;85(1):89–93.

33. Vassileva CM, Markwell S, Boley T, et al. Impact of race on mitral procedure selection and short-term outcomes of patients undergoing mitral valve surgery. Heart Surg Forum 2011;14(4):E221–6.

34. Pienta MJ, Theurer PF, He C, et al. Racial disparities in mitral valve surgery: a statewide analysis. J Thorac Cardiovasc Surg 2022. https://doi.org/10.1016/j.jtcvs.2021.11.096.

35. Beydoun HA, Beydoun MA, Liang H, et al. Sex, race, and socioeconomic disparities in patients with aortic stenosis (from a nationwide inpatient sample). Am J Cardiol 2016;118(6):860–5.

36. Osnabrugge RL, Mylotte D, Head SJ, et al. Aortic stenosis in the elderly: disease prevalence and number of candidates for transcatheter aortic valve replacement: a meta-analysis and modeling study. J Am Coll Cardiol 2013;62(11):1002–12.

37. Singh JP, Evans JC, Levy D, et al. Prevalence and clinical determinants of mitral, tricuspid, and aortic regurgitation (the Framingham Heart Study). Am J Cardiol 1999;83(6):897–902.

38. Patel DK, Green KD, Fudim M, et al. Racial differences in the prevalence of severe aortic stenosis. J Am Heart Assoc 2014;3(3):e000879.

39. Wilson JB, Jackson LR 2nd, Ugowe FE, et al. Racial and ethnic differences in treatment and outcomes of severe aortic stenosis: a review. JACC Cardiovasc Interv 2020;13(2):149–56.

40. Chandra S, Lang RM, Nicolarsen J, et al. Bicuspid aortic valve: inter-racial difference in frequency and aortic dimensions. JACC Cardiovasc Imaging 2012; 5(10):981–9.

41. Stewart BF, Siscovick D, Lind BK, et al. Clinical factors associated with calcific aortic valve disease. Cardiovascular Health Study. J Am Coll Cardiol 1997;29(3):630–4.

42. Cao J, Steffen BT, Budoff M, et al. Lipoprotein(a) levels are associated with subclinical calcific aortic valve disease in white and black individuals: the multi-ethnic study of atherosclerosis. Arterioscler Thromb Vasc Biol 2016;36(5):1003–9.

43. Leon MB, Smith CR, Mack MJ, et al. Transcatheter or surgical aortic-valve replacement in intermediate-risk patients. N Engl J Med 2016;374(17):1609–20.

44. Mack MJ, Leon MB, Thourani VH, et al. Transcatheter aortic-valve replacement with a balloon-expandable valve in low-risk patients. N Engl J Med 2019;380(18):1695–705.

45. Mack MJ, Lindenfeld J, Abraham WT, et al. 3-year outcomes of transcatheter mitral valve repair in patients with heart failure. J Am Coll Cardiol 2021; 77(8):1029–40.

46. Smith CR, Leon MB, Mack MJ, et al. Transcatheter versus surgical aortic-valve replacement in high-risk patients. N Engl J Med 2011;364(23):2187–98.

47. Sleder A, Tackett S, Cerasale M, et al. Socioeconomic and racial disparities: a case-control study of patients receiving transcatheter aortic valve replacement for severe aortic stenosis. J Racial Ethn Health Disparities 2017;4(6):1189–94.

48. Cook NL, Ayanian JZ, Orav EJ, et al. Differences in specialist consultations for cardiovascular disease by race, ethnicity, gender, insurance status, and site of primary care. Circulation 2009;119(18):2463–70.

49. Breathett K, Liu WG, Allen LA, et al. African Americans are less likely to receive care by a cardiologist during an intensive care unit admission for heart failure. JACC Heart Failure 2018;6(5):413–20.

50. Cruz Rodriguez B, Acharya P, Salazar-Fields C, et al. Comparison of frequency of referral to cardiothoracic surgery for aortic valve disease in Blacks, Hispanics, and whites. Am J Cardiol 2017;120(3):450–5.

51. Barreto-Filho JA, Wang Y, Dodson JA, et al. Trends in aortic valve replacement for elderly patients in the United States, 1999-2011. JAMA 2013;310(19):2078–85.

52. Czarny MJ, Hasan RK, Post WS, et al. Inequities in aortic stenosis and aortic valve replacement between Black/African-American, white, and Hispanic residents of Maryland. J Am Heart Assoc 2021; 10(14):e017487.

53. Yankey GS Jr, Jackson LR 2nd, Marts C, et al. African American-Caucasian American differences in aortic valve replacement in patients with severe aortic stenosis. Am Heart J 2021;234:111–21.

54. Taylor NE, O'Brien S, Edwards FH, et al. Relationship between race and mortality and morbidity after valve replacement surgery. Circulation 2005;111(10):1305–12.

55. Alkhouli M, Holmes DR Jr, Carroll JD, et al. Racial disparities in the utilization and outcomes of TAVR: TVT registry report. JACC Cardiovasc Interv 2019; 12(10):936–48.

56. Alkhouli M, Alqahtani F, Holmes DR, et al. Racial disparities in the utilization and outcomes of structural heart disease interventions in the United States. J Am Heart Assoc 2019;8(15):e012125.

57. Gillum RF, Gillum BS, Francis CK. Coronary revascularization and cardiac catheterization in the United States: trends in racial differences. J Am Coll Cardiol 1997;29(7):1557–62.

58. Peterson ED, Shaw LK, DeLong ER, et al. Racial variation in the use of coronary-revascularization procedures. Are the differences real? Do they matter? N Engl J Med 1997;336(7):480–6.

59. Laouri M, Kravitz RL, French WJ, et al. Underuse of coronary revascularization procedures: application of a clinical method. J Am Coll Cardiol 1997;29(5):891–7.

60. Prihadi EA, van der Bijl P, Gursoy E, et al. Development of significant tricuspid regurgitation over time and prognostic implications: new insights into natural history. Eur Heart J 2018;39(39):3574–81.

61. Nath J, Foster E, Heidenreich PA. Impact of tricuspid regurgitation on long-term survival. J Am Coll Cardiol 2004;43(3):405–9.

62. Topilsky Y, Maltais S, Medina Inojosa J, et al. Burden of tricuspid regurgitation in patients diagnosed in the community setting. JACC Cardiovasc Imaging 2019;12(3):433–42.

63. Topilsky Y. Tricuspid valve regurgitation: epidemiology and pathophysiology. Minerva Cardioangiol 2018;66(6):673–9.

64. Vieitez JM, Monteagudo JM, Mahia P, et al. New insights of tricuspid regurgitation: a large-scale prospective cohort study. Eur Heart J Cardiovasc Imaging 2021;22(2):196–202.

65. Condello F, Gitto M, Stefanini GG. Etiology, epidemiology, pathophysiology and management of tricuspid regurgitation: an overview. Rev Cardiovasc Med 2021;22(4):1115–42.

66. Aluru JS, Barsouk A, Saginala K, et al. Valvular heart disease epidemiology. Med Sci 2022;10(2). https://doi.org/10.3390/medsci10020032.

67. Rodés-Cabau J, Taramasso M, O'Gara PT. Diagnosis and treatment of tricuspid valve disease: current and future perspectives. Lancet 2016;388(10058):2431–42.

68. Alqahtani F, Berzingi CO, Aljohani S, et al. Contemporary trends in the use and outcomes of surgical treatment of tricuspid regurgitation. J Am Heart Assoc 2017;6(12). https://doi.org/10.1161/JAHA.117.007597.

69. Pfannmueller B, Eifert S, Seeburger J, et al. Gender-dependent differences in patients undergoing tricuspid valve surgery. Thorac Cardiovasc Surg 2013;61(1):37–41.

70. Fam NP, von Bardeleben RS, Hensey M, et al. Transfemoral transcatheter tricuspid valve replacement with the EVOQUE system: a multicenter, observational, first-in-human experience. JACC Cardiovasc Interv 2021;14(5):501–11.

71. Sedhom R, Megaly M, Saad M, et al. Transcatheter edge-to-edge repair of the tricuspid valve: the US experience. Catheter Cardiovasc Interv 2022;99(6): 1859–66.

72. Lurz P, Stephan von Bardeleben R, Weber M, et al. Transcatheter edge-to-edge repair for treatment of tricuspid regurgitation. J Am Coll Cardiol 2021; 77(3):229–39.

73. Tsao CW, Aday AW, Almarzooq ZI, et al. Heart disease and stroke statistics-2022 update: a report from the American Heart Association. Circulation 2022;145(8):e153–639.

74. Choong CY, Abascal VM, Weyman J, et al. Prevalence of valvular regurgitation by Doppler echocardiography in patients with structurally normal hearts by two-dimensional echocardiography. Am Heart J 1989;117(3):636–42.

75. Heery E, Sheehan AM, While AE, et al. Experiences and outcomes of transition from pediatric to adult health care services for young people with congenital heart disease: a systematic review. Congenit Heart Dis 2015;10(5):413–27.

76. Mazurenko O, Balio CP, Agarwal R, et al. The effects of Medicaid expansion under the ACA: a systematic review. Health Aff 2018;37(6):944–50.

77. Breathett KK, Xu H, Sweitzer NK, et al. Is the affordable care act Medicaid expansion associated with receipt of heart failure guideline-directed medical therapy by race and ethnicity? Am Heart J 2022; 244:135–48.

78. Breathett K, Allen LA, Helmkamp L, et al. The affordable care act Medicaid expansion correlated with increased heart transplant listings in African Americans but not Hispanics or Caucasians. JACC Heart Failure 2017;5(2):136–47.

79. Warner JJ, Benjamin IJ, Churchwell K, et al. Advancing healthcare reform: the American Heart Association's 2020 statement of principles for adequate, accessible, and affordable health care: a presidential advisory from the American Heart Association. Circulation 2020;141(10):e601–14.

80. D'Agostino RS, Jacobs JP, Badhwar V, et al. The Society of Thoracic Surgeons adult cardiac surgery database: 2017 update on outcomes and quality. Ann Thorac Surg 2017;103(1):18–24.

81. Balady GJ, Ades PA, Bittner VA, et al. Referral, enrollment, and delivery of cardiac rehabilitation/secondary prevention programs at clinical centers and beyond: a presidential advisory from the American Heart Association. Circulation 2011;124(25): 2951–60.

82. Sullivan LT, Randolph T, Merrill P, et al. Representation of black patients in randomized clinical trials of heart failure with reduced ejection fraction. Am Heart J 2018;197:43–52.

83. Reza N, Gruen J, Bozkurt B. Representation of women in heart failure clinical trials: barriers to enrollment and strategies to close the gap. Am Heart J 2022;13. https://doi.org/10.1016/j.ahjo.2022.100093.

84. Scott PE, Unger EF, Jenkins MR, et al. Participation of women in clinical trials supporting FDA approval of cardiovascular drugs. J Am Coll Cardiol 2018; 71(18):1960–9.

85. Whitelaw S, Thabane L, Mamas MA, et al. Characteristics of heart failure trials associated with underrepresentation of women as lead authors. J Am Coll Cardiol 2020;76(17):1919–30.

86. Clark LT, Watkins L, Pina IL, et al. Increasing diversity in clinical trials: overcoming critical barriers. Curr Probl Cardiol 2019;44(5):148–72.

87. Ilonze OJ, Avorgbedor F, Diallo A, et al. Addressing challenges faced by underrepresented biomedical investigators and efforts to address them: an NHLBI-PRIDE perspective. J Natl Med Assoc 2022. https://doi.org/10.1016/j.jnma.2022.09.007.

88. Oh SS, Galanter J, Thakur N, et al. Diversity in clinical and biomedical research: a promise yet to be fulfilled. PLoS Med 2015;12(12):e1001918.

89. Morris AA, Khazanie P, Drazner MH, et al. Guidance for timely and appropriate referral of patients with advanced heart failure: a scientific statement from the American Heart Association. Circulation 2021; 144(15):e238–50.

90. Breathett K, Yee E, Pool N, et al. Does race influence decision making for advanced heart failure therapies? J Am Heart Assoc 2019;8(22):e013592.

91. Thornton RL, Powe NR, Roter D, et al. Patient-physician social concordance, medical visit communication and patients' perceptions of health care quality. Patient Educ Couns 2011;85(3):e201–8.

92. Jackson JL, Kay C, Scholcoff C, et al. Associations between gender and racial patient-physician concordance and visit outcomes among hypertensive patients in primary care. J Gen Intern Med 2022;37(6): 1569–71.

93. Arendt F, Karadas N. Ethnic concordance in patient-physician communication: experimental evidence from Germany. J Health Commun 2019;24(1):1–8.

94. Perez-Stable EJ, El-Toukhy S. Communicating with diverse patients: how patient and clinician factors affect disparities. Patient Educ Couns 2018;101(12):2186–94.

95. Stout KK, Daniels CJ, Aboulhosn JA, et al. 2018 AHA/ACC guideline for the management of adults with congenital heart disease: a report of the American College of Cardiology/American Heart Association

Task Force on Clinical Practice Guidelines. J Am Coll Cardiol 2019;73(12):e81–192.

96. Promotion OoDPaH. Social determinants of health. Healthy people 2030. U.S. Department of Health and Human Services. 2021. Available at: https://health.gov/healthypeople/objectives-and-data/social-determinants-health.

97. Churchwell K, Elkind MSV, Benjamin RM, et al. Call to action: structural racism as a fundamental driver of health disparities: a presidential advisory from the american heart association. Circulation 2020; 142(24):e454–68.

98. Lewsey SC, Breathett K. Racial and ethnic disparities in heart failure: current state and future directions. Curr Opin Cardiol 2021;36(3):320–8.

The Emerging Role of Artificial Intelligence in Valvular Heart Disease

Caroline Canning, MSc, MBI[a,b], James Guo[a,b], Akhil Narang, MD[a,b], James D. Thomas, MD[a,b], Faraz S. Ahmad, MD, MS[a,b,c],*

KEYWORDS

- Valvular heart disease • Artificial intelligence • Machine learning • Deep learning
- Natural language processing • Heart failure

KEY POINTS

- Valvular heart disease is a morbid condition with several unmet needs.
- Machine learning has the potential to improve the care of patients with valvular heart disease by facilitating screening, improving severity classification, identifying phenogroups, and improving risk prediction.
- Applications of machine learning in valvular heart disease are early in development and require additional testing.

INTRODUCTION

Valvular heart disease (VHD) has been found in 14% of patients referred for echocardiographic workup of suspected heart failure (HF)[1] and 21% of patients hospitalized for HF.[2] The epidemiology of VHD varies around the world. In high-income countries, VHD is predominantly due to degenerative disease, whereas in low-income and middle-income countries, VHD is predominantly due to rheumatic heart disease.[3] Even with this variance, the global incidence of VHD has increased by 45% in the last 30 years due to an aging population,[4] contributing to burden of degenerative disease.[4,5] Consequently, the proportion of HF secondary to VHD is likely to increase.[3] Aortic and mitral valvulopathies predominate in prevalence, particularly calcific aortic valve disease and degenerative mitral valve disease.[1,3] Substantial advances in the management of severe VHD have been made in recent decades with the development of transcatheter approaches to valve repair and replacement. Transcatheter aortic and mitral valve procedures have increased by nearly 5-fold and 10-fold, respectively, in recent years with growing favorable outcomes.[6,7] Tricuspid transcatheter valve repair and replacement are also emerging therapies and are currently under investigation.[8,9]

VHD is a ripe area for the development and testing of artificial intelligence (AI) or machine learning (ML) approaches. A systematic review of AI/ML in cardiovascular medicine found that less than 3% of studies were applied in this disease area.[10] Cardiovascular medicine is increasingly digital, with widespread integration of electronic health records (EHRs) in clinical practice, repositories of cardiovascular diagnostic data including echocardiograms, electrocardiogram (ECG), phonocardiograms (PCGs), and cardiac computed tomography (CT) and MRI. The vast amount of data

[a] Division of Cardiology, Department of Medicine, Northwestern University Feinberg School of Medicine, 676 North St. Clair Street, Suite 600, Chicago, IL 60611, USA; [b] Bluhm Cardiovascular Institute Center for Artificial Intelligence, Northwestern Medicine, Chicago, IL, USA; [c] Division of Health and Biomedical informatics, Department of Preventive Medicine, Northwestern University Feinberg School of Medicine, Chicago, IL, USA
* Corresponding author.
E-mail address: faraz.ahmad@northwestern.edu
Twitter: @carolinecanning (C.C.); @AkhilNarangMD (A.N.); @jamesdthomasMD1 (J.D.T.); @FarazAhmadMD (F.S.A.)

Heart Failure Clin 19 (2023) 391–405
https://doi.org/10.1016/j.hfc.2023.03.001
1551-7136/23/© 2023 Elsevier Inc. All rights reserved.

coupled with the increased availability of high-performance computing will be conducive to the continued growth in AI and ML research and application development to improve detection, risk prediction, and management of VHD.

AI broadly refers to the ability for computers to perform tasks and problem solve like the human mind. ML is a subset of AI that emerged from the fields of computer science and statistics. ML relies on input, specifically large collections of data, to recognize patterns, entities, and the connections between them. The discipline of ML explores the analysis and construction of algorithms that can learn from and make predictions based on data. ML algorithms build a mathematical model based on sample data, known as training data, to make predictions or decisions without being explicitly programmed to do so.[11] An increasingly utilized subset of ML is deep learning (DL), or artificial neural networks (ANNs). This specifically refers to algorithms that are modeled after the human brain containing artificial "neurons" arranged in successive layers culminating in a decision function. This relationship is illustrated in **Fig. 1**.

Typically, an ML dataset will be split into 3 categories: training, validation, and testing. The training subset is used to fit an ML model. The validation subset is to test the model and tweak certain hyperparameters because it is trained to optimize performance. Finally, the test subset is used to evaluate the fit, or model performance of the ML model. It is important that the test subset be segregated from the rest of the data so it cannot be included in the training and validation.

Two main approaches, supervised and unsupervised learning, have been widely applied to a variety of clinical problems and tasks in biomedical science. Supervised learning requires human input to label input and output training data. A model will learn the relationship between the inputs and outputs, and will adjust to make the correct answer. Therefore, supervised models are generally used for classification or regression (predicting outcomes). Unsupervised learning identifies intrinsic patterns within data without human intervention, and the output of the model is generally patterns or trends. These models generally include clustering, association tasks, dimensionality reduction, or factorization. Unsupervised learning can be used in exploratory data analysis to inform supervised learning tasks. Other types of learning frameworks, such as reinforcement learning, have been applied in health care. Several reviews have described in detail different ML approaches, applications, strengths, and limitations for addressing problems in health care more broadly and within cardiovascular medicine.[10,12–17]

In this review, we highlight areas AI/ML methods and their application may address the following unmet needs in the care of patients with VHD: (1) screening for VHD, (2) assessment of severity of disease, (3) risk prediction, and (4) phenomapping (**Fig. 2**). Later, we discuss some of the challenges and future directions of AI/ML in VHD.

SCREENING FOR VALVULAR HEART DISEASE

Several studies have shown that VHD remains underdiagnosed.[18–22] In the United States alone, national prevalence of VHD affects 2.5% of the population.[19] Most patients are not screened for VHD until they report the onset of symptoms even though most cases remain asymptomatic for many years.[19,22] This presents an opportunity for early detection before the lesion becomes more severe, causes symptoms, or leads to ventricular dilation or dysfunction. More studies are calling for early identification and treatment of VHD,[23,24] and thus timely identification has implications for disease management and improvement of patient outcomes.[25–27] The gold standard of detecting VHD is via echocardiogram[18] but due to cost and resource limitations it is usually reserved for either symptomatic patients or those for whom there is high clinical suspicion of VHD based on physical examination. Other cardiac examinations that are more widely indicated can help recognize patients with asymptomatic VHD that should be referred for an echo. Below we explore examples of studies that are using ML strategies to help identify patients with VHD through auscultation and ECG. Although these examples show that these technologies can identify patients with underdiagnosed VHD, prospective randomized controlled trials and cost-effectiveness analyses are needed to inform recommendations from guideline-writing organizations, such as various cardiovascular societies and the US Preventive Services Task Force.

Auscultation

The stethoscope was invented in 1818 by René Laennec. It has remained the most inexpensive and accessible modality to detect VHD as heart sounds can reveal the cause of a lesion as well as the severity. Although every clinician learns to auscultate as a foundational part of the physical examination, the ability to detect and interpret murmurs varies widely.[28,29] Thus, researchers have explored ways to aid clinicians in this task.

Attempts to classify pathologic condition in PCGs, or visual plot representation of heart sounds, has been performed for more than

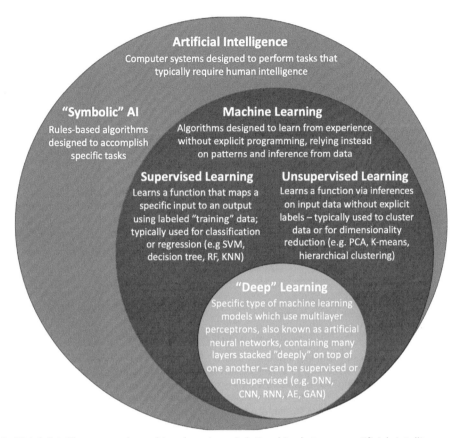

Fig. 1. Artificial intelligence and machine learning. Relationship between artificial intelligence, machine learning, and "deep" learning. CNN, convolutional neural network; DNN, deep neural network; GAN, generative adversarial network; KNN, k-nearest neighbor; PCA, principal components analysis; RF, random forests; RNN, recurrent neural network; SVM, Support vector machines; VAE, variational autoencoder. (*From* Wehbe RM, Khan SS, Shah SJ, Ahmad FS. Predicting High-Risk Patients and High-Risk Outcomes in Heart Failure. Heart Fail Clin. 2020;16(4):387-407.)

50 years. This was accelerated by the 2016 PhysioNet/Computing in Cardiology Challenge,[30] which published an open-access database of 3126 heart sound recordings. Researchers were tasked with identifying PCGs as normal, abnormal, or poor signal quality. The 3 top performing entrants used ensemble methods, or combination of different classifiers to improve accuracy. However, each team used different classifiers, demonstrating that different approaches could have comparable performance.[31] The feature extraction stage, which transforms the data into derived values, or features, to reduce redundancy was deemed key to effective models.[31]

Digital stethoscopes have enabled the recording and automated classification of heart sounds. These stethoscopes work by converting acoustic sound to electronic signals, which can be amplified for the examiner.[32] Many models can transmit the information to a mobile app or computer in the form of an audio file or PCG.[32]

One AI-enabled digital stethoscope that detects and characterizes murmurs in adults and pediatric patients has received Food and Drug Administration (FDA) clearance and Conformite Europeenne (CE) mark. This was supported by a study from Chorba and colleagues,[33] who created and tested a deep convolutional neural network (CNN) model that classifies PCGs in 3 categories: heart murmur, no murmur, or inadequate signal. To determine the accuracy of the signal quality and murmur detection performance, the algorithm output was compared with annotations from 3 cardiologists. Algorithm performance had a sensitivity and specificity for detecting murmurs of 76.3% and 91.4%. The study also used the gold standard echocardiogram to detect "clinically significant" (more than moderate) aortic stenosis (AS) and mitral regurgitation (MR). Detection of AS at the aortic position was 93.2% sensitive and 86.0% specific. The detection of MR at the mitral position was 66.2% sensitive and 94.6% specific.

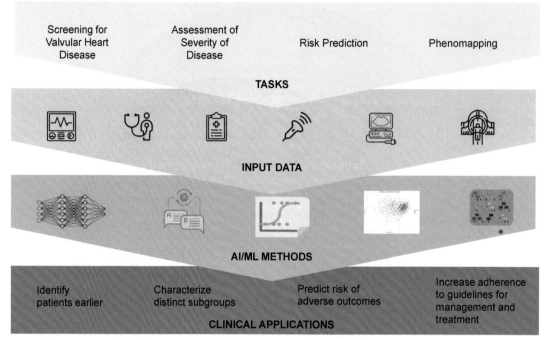

Fig. 2. Clinical applications of AI/ML in valvular heart disease. Four main tasks for AI/ML in valvular heart disease are reviewed in this article: (1) screening to valvular heart disease, (2) assessment of severity of disease, (3) risk prediction, and (4) phenomapping. For each task, a variety of data types and models have been applied, predominantly in retrospective datasets. Each of these has the potential to lead to improvements in clinical care in 4 main areas but additional, prospective clinical studies are needed.

Electrocardiogram

Besides auscultation, ECG is another relatively inexpensive and ubiquitous noninvasive test to evaluate the heart. In current clinical practice, valvular diseases are not directly diagnosed on ECG but evidence of structural heart disease, such as left ventricular hypertrophy, can provide clues for VHD leading to left ventricular remodeling. Several studies have examined whether DL can be applied to ECGs to detect VHD in patients.

The ability to detect and predict the future development of severe AS is of interest because the condition is associated with a mortality rate of 40% to 50% within 1 year without valve replacement.[34,35] Multiple groups of investigators have trained a specific neural network called a CNN, which are often used for image classification and process an image in a grid-like fashion, using ECG-Echo pairs. Kwon and colleagues[36] used 39,371 ECGs from patients at a cardiology teaching hospital to train a CNN to detect AS, and then performed external validation on the algorithm with 10,865 ECGs from patients at a community hospital, which showed generalizability with an area under the curve (AUC) of 0.861, sensitivity 0.80, and specificity 0.78. They also used a

saliency map, which focused on the T wave, to highlight the parts of the ECG that were used to predict presence of AS. This type of technique has been used to increase confidence for clinicians to accept the prediction results because the user sees that the algorithm is using an important feature to make a prediction rather than some artifact in the background. Results from Cohen Shelley and colleagues[37] reinforce these findings. The authors trained a CNN to identify moderate-to-severe AS in 258,607 adults with ECG-TTE pairs, with a comparable AUC of 0.85, sensitivity of 0.78, and specificity of 0.74 when using just ECG morphology alone. Their saliency map similarly highlighted the TP segment as an area of importance. However, several studies have raised concerns about the accuracy and reliability of saliency maps for DL algorithms and emphasize the need for prospective testing of algorithms to generate the evidence base to support adoption over the reliance of saliency maps and other techniques to increase confidence of end-users.[38,39]

Because the overall incidence of VHD is relatively low, the rECHOmmend study[40] combined moderate-to-severe valvular disease (AS, AR, MS, MR, tricuspid regurgitation [TR]) with structural changes of reduced EF less than 50%, or ventricular septal thickness greater than 15 mm to achieve increased positive predictive value (PPV) for their models. Authors marked ECGs as positive for a given condition if it was acquired within a year before the patient's first positive echocardiogram for the label. Then they trained a CNN to predict presence or absence of any of the 7 labels with ECG tracings and a range of input data including demographics, laboratories, findings, and ECG measurements. Although the model performed best with all inputs, the area under the receiver operating characteristic (AUROC) remained high (0.91) with age, sex, and ECG tracing data. This potentially enables more targeted referral for echocardiography to help detect underdiagnosed VHD, although prospective testing is needed to determine the clinical utility and cost-effectiveness of these approaches.

ASSESSMENT OF SEVERITY FOR VALVULAR HEART DISEASE

The studies that explore severity predominantly use echocardiography as an input, as echocardiography remains the primary modality for diagnosis and evaluation of VHD.[18] Echocardiograms are one of the least expensive and most accessible forms of cardiac imaging.[41–43] Between 2001 and 2011, there were more than 7 million echocardiograms performed annually in the United States, with its use increasing by more than 3% yearly.[41] AI has been used for a variety of tasks related to echocardiography,[44–47] including view acquisition, view classification,[48] quality assessment,[49] automation of measurements and observations,[50,51] and disease identification, such as cardiac amyloidosis[52] and hypertrophic cardiomyopathy.[53–55]

The use of AI to diagnose VHDs via echocardiographic images represents an emerging area of research. For example, Yang and colleagues[56] developed a 3-stage DL framework that evaluated view classification, screening for VHDs (aortic and mitral lesions), and when positive, performed segmentation to provide metrics related to severity. The investigators used 2 different approaches to detect regurgitant and stenotic lesions. A CNN was trained to detect color in the left ventricular outflow tract (LVOT) or left atrium for AR and MR, respectively. It also measured anatomic structures to localize the regurgitation in time and space. For stenotic lesions, the algorithm identified the PLAX-2D and A4C views as input for the diagnosis and then calculated valve area with Doppler to calculate mitral stenosis (MS), and the Vmax and mean pressure gradients for AS. Overall, the DL model provided varying agreement when compared with measurements by 2 physician echocardiographers with Intersection of Union (IoU) metrics. IoU is also referred to as the Jaccard Index, is a common metric used in image segmentation. The lowest IoU was for AR jet 0.63, whereas the highest IoU was for the left atrial area 0.86. Next, the model achieved high performance for identifying valvular stenosis and regurgitation with AUC for MS 0.95, MR 0.97, AS 0.91, and AR 0.97 using retrospective data. Finally, the study concluded that the accuracy of the degree of valve lesion severity was within the bounds of normal practice when compared with 2 experienced physicians. They also validated their results in prospective, consecutive cases (n=1374) to demonstrate generalizability and adequate performance outside of the dataset used for training. This study describes in detail the development and testing of a pipeline for a complex set of tasks and posted their code in a public repository, both of which are essential to promoting reproducibility and advances in this field.

In a study by Sengupta and colleagues,[57] used both unsupervised and supervised ML classifiers to predict high-severity or low-severity AS. Their model was trained on echocardiographic data from 1052 patients with AS and derived high-severity and low-severity groups of AS, they validated their association of severity with other markers of AS such as AV calcium score on CT, markers of myocardial damage on CMR, and biomarkers such as brain natriuretic peptide (BNP). The ML model was able to correctly classify 99% of patients with definitive echocardiographic features of severe AS into the high-severity group. Notably, it was also able to reclassify the remaining patients with either nonsevere AS or inconclusive discordant echocardiographic findings without additional tests. When compared with conventional strategies for AS severity classification, the ML severity classification improved discrimination (integrated discrimination improvement: 0.07; 95% CI: 0.02–0.12) and reclassification (net reclassification improvement: 0.17; 95% CI: 0.11–0.23) for the outcome of aortic valve replacement (AVR) at 5 years. The investigators show that ML can analyze echocardiographic measurements to accurately classify AS severity in most patients with potential to optimize timing of AVR.

Recent preliminary results from a commercial AI-echo company sought to detect and characterize aortic stenosis purely from B-mode images without spectral or color Doppler. Trained on 30,000 echoes (parasternal long axis and short axis and apical 5-chamber views), a test set demonstrated detection of moderate-or-severe

AS with sensitivity of 91% and specificity of 94%.[58] Another commercial AI company developed the ability to identify severe AS with clinical characteristics and echocardiogram measurements without LVOT data. The model performed equally independent of AS gradients.[59] An increasing number of companies are developing technology in this space and will be subject to FDA review.

In addition to classifying VHD severity, AI can be used to acquisition of images by personnel without earlier ultrasound experience to obtain diagnostic quality echoes.[60] With further development and validation for the destination of VHD, this use case of AI could be scaled to resource-limited settings without access to trained sonographers to better detect conditions such as rheumatic heart disease.

Besides using echocardiogram images and videos, natural language processing (NLP) has been used to extract valve severity from echocardiogram reports given the challenges with capturing and using structured data generated by echocardiographers and the limited accuracy of International Classification of Diseases (ICD) coding.[61,62] NLP can be rule-based or use ML. Solomon and colleagues[61] developed an NLP algorithm with the goal of making sure that all patients with VHD are appropriately followed. The NLP algorithm had a 99% PPV and 99% NPV for identifying prevalent AS. They found that among those classified as having AS by the NLP, only 64.6% of patients had an ICD diagnosis code of AS. They also found that the NLP-derived hemodynamic parameters were concordant with the physician designated levels of severity. Identifying and recording a patient's diagnosis in the medical record and developing care pathways can help increase rates of appropriate follow-up in accordance to clinical guidelines.[18]

Another strategy to make sure a diagnosis is not missed is through clinical decision support (CDS). CDS are tools embedded in a clinical workflow, such as the EHR, to help improve decision-making. A multicenter study of 35 institutions used 1,147,157 echocardiograms to build a tool to help identify patients who may mistakenly not have received a diagnosis of severe AS called the Diagnostic Precision Algorithm.[63] The tool uses echocardiographic parameters to determine if patients with similar measurements would be likely to have severe AS, then it prioritizes patients for review based on how likely these valve measurements would be considered severe. The NLP is used to detect that the echocardiogram report was not categorized as severe AS. Overall, the Diagnostic Precision Algorithm was able to predict the proportion of severe AS versus the actual proportion with an average error of 2.1% in the prediction model with left ventricular ejection fraction (LVEF) and an error of 2.2% without LVEF. As the authors highlight, the algorithm demonstrated high accuracy and yields good potential for application to assist physicians to follow-up with patients with potentially undiagnosed severe AS.[18]

Alternatively to clinician CDS, similar to HF, workflows could be created to either support a population health approach in which a member of the clinical team reviews cases and works with the patients' primary team to ensure adherence to guideline recommends or directly nudge the patient to discuss evidence-based care for VHD with their clinician.[64,65]

RISK PREDICTION

Risk prediction models are equations that use patient risk factors to estimate the probability of a health-care outcome. Well-known risk-prediction models include the Well's Criteria[66] for pulmonary embolism or the Quick SOFA (qSOFA) score[67] for identifying high-risk mortality from sepsis in critically ill patients. ML is just one tool among many that can be used to create these models. In VHD, ML has been applied largely in the area of predicting outcomes and response to AVR rather than determining the risk of developing VHD.

The discrepancy of the aortic valve area and low transvalvular gradient makes the management of patients with low gradient AS challenging.[68] Namasivayam and colleagues[69] developed the Aortic Stenosis Risk (ASteRisk) with the goal of predicting outcomes within 5 years of follow-up for patients with moderate-to-severe AS that would be interpretable and also effective in patients with low-gradient AS. Using bootstrap Lasso regression (Least Absolute Shrinkage and Selection Operator), they selected a subset of variables for a logistic regression model that minimized prediction error (AUC = 0.74). They limited the ASteRisk score to include 9 readily available variables that include a mix of echocardiogram measurements and clinical history to maximize the ease of use in practice. Some of the risk factors included aortic valve area, mean gradient, energy loss, HF, hyperlipidemia, and CKD. They found the ASteRisk model superior to predicting all-cause mortality or AVR in moderate-to-severe AS patients for years 2 to 5, versus a baseline model that used more conventional risk factors (mean transvalvular gradient, aortic valve area, age, and LVEF). The model also worked in patients with low-gradient AS. They tested generalizability on patients from another institution that identified patients at high risk of death at 1 to 5 years. Additional external validation and, ideally, prospective testing, will help elucidate the clinical usefulness of this model for clinical decision-making.

CMR can provide information about not only the structure and function of the heart but also the degree of myocardial fibrosis.[70] Kwak and colleagues set out to investigate if how markers of damage on CMR could predict prognosis in severe AS and help guide timing for AVR.[71] Investigators used a supervised ML method called Random Forest, a technique that outputs the average result of multiple decision trees, to determine the predictors of death in patients with severe AS undergoing AVR. The study used clinical, echocardiogram, and CMR variables but remained focused on 4 CMR variables, which emerged as most predictive of all cause mortality: extracellular volume fraction (ECV%), late gadolinium enhancement (LGE%), right ventricular ejection fraction (RVEF), and indexed left ventricular end-diastolic volume (LVEDVi). They analyzed the parameters of each variable associated with markedly worse prognosis and built an AS-CMR risk score, in which a point was given for ECV% greater than 27%, REVF 50 or lesser or greater than 80%, LGE% greater than 2%, and LVEDVi 55 or lesser or greater than 80 mL/m². Noting the importance of RVEF as an important prognostic marker, authors posited that these patients may benefit from TAVR, where RV function is generally maintained, versus SAVR, which is associated with RV dysfunction after surgery.

PHENOMAPPING

Many have posited that ML will be a critical tool in achieving personalized medicine, where medical decisions are tailored to an individual's phenotype. VHDs, even of the same severity, are heterogenous syndromes similar to other cardiovascular conditions. ML methods have been used in multiple studies to define phenogroups, or groups of patients with similar clinical characteristics, and differential risk of adverse outcomes.

In aortic stenosis, valve area, transaortic gradient, and maximum aortic velocity are the primary quantitative measurements to stratify severity. One study of patients with severe aortic stenosis used 3 unsupervised, independent methods to identify 4 phenogroups.[72] Then, the investigators used a supervised algorithm to predict survival outcomes by each cluster. Each group had an increased amount of myocardial damage and mortality, regardless of the severity of AS. Therefore, authors concluded cardiac remodeling and progression of systolic and diastolic dysfunction plays a large role in prognosis. Guidelines recommend patients with symptomatic, severe AS undergoing evaluation for aortic valve replacement[18] but these results suggest cardiac remodeling may be another factor during the evaluation for timing of intervention in asymptomatic patients.[72]

Several other studies of AS have used unsupervised methods to identify clusters with different rates of adverse events after valve replacement. Lachmann and colleagues[73] used unsupervised clustering among patients undergoing TAVR for severe AS, identifying 4 clusters with variations of pulmonary hypertension, LVEF, and prevalence of other valvular defects. Then, investigators tested the ability to reproduce the phenogroups prospectively by categorizing the patients into clusters with an ANN, following their clinical course, and measuring the different rates of adverse events between groups. Kwak and colleagues[74] grouped 398 patients with moderate-to-severe AS into 3 clusters that were broadly defined as patients with (1) cardiac dysfunction, (2) comorbidities (particularly ESRD), and (3) healthy AS with neither cardiac dysfunction nor comorbidities. Although AS severity between clusters did not differ, mortality rate was significantly different between clusters. During a median 2.4-year follow-up, the comorbidities cluster had the highest mortality rate of 19.8% versus the healthy AS cluster had the lowest mortality rate of 6.0% during the 2.4 years.

Phenomapping has also produced valuable insights about MR. There are many causes of secondary MR.[75] Bartko and colleagues[76] focused on phenomapping in sMR in patients with HF with reduced ejection fraction (HFrEF) using echocardiogram measurements and clinical variables. Principal component analysis, which is an unsupervised learning technique for dimensionality reduction, identifies the most informative variables in the data. Investigators found 4 phenogroups with different morphologies of varying LV and LA size and dilation. Each cluster had stepwise progression in sMR severity but regurgitant fraction peaked in Cluster 3, which was characterized by small LV and extensive LA dilation. The approach suggested that clinicians should consider not only LV remodeling but also LA and mitral valve annulus. Notably, authors published a simplified calculator that clinicians can use to identify which cluster an individual patient belongs to. Further translating these phenogroups into practice, the investigators remarked that these phenotypes may help explain difference in outcome from 2 landmark MitraClip (Abbot Laboratories) clinical trials, and the need to better understand patient selection and MR phenogroups.[77,78]

The 2020 ACC/AHA Guidelines for Management of Patients with Valvular Heart Disease noted thresholds for interventions are expanding because of randomized clinical trials.[18] Whether phenogroup mapping will provide clinically meaningful information and ultimately inform the decision-making process for valvular interventions remain unanswered questions.

DISCUSSION

We have discussed some of the unmet needs in the early detection, diagnosis, and management of VHD that may be addressed by AI-enabled technologies. Examples include screening for VHD with ECG or PCG, improving the classification of the severity of specific types of VHD, and phenomapping and risk prediction to identify subgroups at differential risk for worsening disease and cardiovascular events (**Tables 1** and **2**, see **Fig. 2**). Most research currently leverages data from a single modality or multimodal tabular data but a growing area AI and VHD research in the coming years will be developing models leveraging a combination of unstructured and structured, multimodal, longitudinal data.[79] Research will also likely increase training models using self-supervised learning, which has outperformed other DL algorithms for several language tasks and now is being more widely tested in computer vision, signal analytics, and other data types.[14]

Another expanding area of research will be the application of large language models. ChatGPT and BioGPT, released by OpenAI and Microsoft in late 2022, are transformer-based language models that have caught the attention of researchers and lay-people alike but have yet to be applied to VHD research. The application of large language models to VHD and health care more broadly must be taken when using these limitations of these models as noted by the ChatGPT developers: "ChatGPT sometimes writes plausible-sounding but incorrect or nonsensical answers."[80]

The application of AI to VHD remains an emerging area of research and application development. The Food and Drug Administration has 3 specific pathways for the approval of AI/ML-based medical technologies and requires the use of "locked" algorithms—algorithms that remain static over time—for use as part of clinical care.[81] However, beyond FDA approval, often several additional steps are necessary before broader adoption of the AI/ML based medical technology into clinical practice and incorporation into clinical guidelines. For example, the accurate identification of prevalent VHD with ECG or PCG represents an initial step. Prospective clinical trials evaluating the clinical effectiveness and cost-effectiveness of screening strategies are an important step for adoption into clinical guidelines. Furthermore, implementation studies examining barriers and facilitators to and costs of implementation in hospitals and clinics are also essential to broader adoption of these technologies.[82,83] Finally, several factors unrelated to the algorithms themselves (known as dataset shift) can lead to decreased model performance over time.[84] There remains a need for the development of robust governance systems to monitor model performance once deployed into clinical settings.

Strategies to better identify and reduce bias in ML models is an active area of investigation in the ML community. Several studies have shown that ML models can embed aspects of structural racism, gender, and implicit bias into their algorithms and potentially exacerbate health inequities.[85–88] Addressing these biases during the training, testing, and validation of AI/ML technologies for VHD will be critical to realize the potential benefit of these technologies across diverse

Table 1
Artificial intelligence applications included in this review

Valve	Valvulopathy	Screening for VHD	Severity of Disease	Risk Stratification	Phenomapping
Aortic	Stenosis	x	x	x	x
	Regurgitation	x	x		
Mitral	Stenosis	x	x		
	Regurgitation	x	x		x
Tricuspid	Stenosis		Not present		
	Regurgitation	x			
Pulmonary	Stenosis		Not present		
	Regurgitation				

Table 2
Highlighted artificial intelligence/machine learning algorithms in valvular heart disease

Category	Title	Authors	ML Approach	Model Training Data	Objective	Key Findings
Screening for VHD	rECHOmmend: An ECG-Based Machine Learning Approach for Identifying Patients at Increased Risk of Undiagnosed Structural Heart Disease Detectable by Echocardiography	Ulloa-Cerna AE, Jing L, Pfeifer JM, et al.	Convolutional Neural Network with XGBoost	2,925,925 ECGs from 631,710 patients, clinical demographics (age, sex), laboratories, vitals	Detect AS, AR, MS, MR, TR, reduced EF <50% or ventricular septum thickness >15 mm	Model using just ECG tracing, age, sex had AUC = 0.91 at sensitivity 0.90, with a PPV of 0.42 for clinically meaningful disease. Validated at 10 other sites, with AUCs 0.79–0.93
Severity of Disease	Automated Analysis of Doppler Echocardiographic Videos as a Screening Tool for Valvular Heart Diseases	Yang Feifei, Chen Xiaotian, Lin Xixiang, et al.	Convolutional Neural Network	1,335 echocardiogram Doppler videos and images	Echocardiogram view classification, segmentation, identification of stenosis vs regurgitation, and grading of severity	In retrospective dataset for identifying aortic and mitral valve stenosis and regurgitation all accuracy ≥0.87, sensitivities ≥0.82, specificities ≥0.88. For prospective cohort, model performance similar for stenosis, and slightly decreased for regurgitation
Risk Stratification	Markers of Myocardial Damage Predict Mortality in Patients With Aortic Stenosis	Kwak S, Everett RJ, Treibel TA, et al.	Random Survival Forest	CMR measurements, echocardiogram measurements, demographics, clinical variables from 440 patients	Identify markers of myocardial fibrosis in CMR that are prognostic in AS for patients undergoing AVR	Created the AS-CMR score to identify patients at high risk of mortality post-AVR.

(continued on next page)

Table 2
(continued)

Category	Title	Authors	ML Approach	Model Training Data	Objective	Key Findings
						Patient gets one point for ECV % >27%, RVEF ≤50 or >80%, LGE % >2%, LVEDVi ≤55 or >80 mL/m². Each point has statistically significant difference in 3 y mortality
Phenomapping	Principal Morphomic and Functional Components of Secondary Mitral Regurgitation	Bartko PE, Heitzinger G, Spinka G, et al.	Principal Component Analysis	Morphology and functional parameters from echocardiograms (32 variables) from 383 patients	Identify different phenogroups of secondary MR patients with HFrEF	Identified four clusters of patients with atrial and ventricular morphologies, and regurgitant fractions. Each cluster had statistically significant survival times. Published an online tool to calculate for individual patient

Abbreviations: AR, aortic regurgitation; AS, aortic stenosis; AVR, aortic valve replacement; CMR, cardiovascular magnetic resonance; ECG, electrocardiogram; ECV%, extracellular volume fraction; EF, ejection fraction; HFrEF, heart failure with reduced ejection fraction; LGE%, late gadolinium enhancement; LVEDVi, indexed left ventricular end-diastolic volume; MR, mitral regurgitation; MS, mitral stenosis; RVEF, right ventricular ejection fraction; TR, tricuspid regurgitation.

populations and as a potential lever to advance equity.

In addition to concerns with biases in algorithms and deprecation in model performance when applied to new populations or over time, the "black box" nature of many algorithms remains a challenge to adoption. This issue is particularly salient in cardiovascular imaging as CNNs, which are black box algorithms, are widely used in studies. Although some clinicians may remain skeptical of AI-enabled technologies without the use of methods to identify the primary features contributing to a prediction, several experts have demonstrated the limitations of these methods.[38,39] Ultimately, similar to medications, the mechanism of action may be less important in the presence of high-quality evidence of benefit generated by randomized controlled trials.[38]

Guidelines are emerging to promote transparency in reporting and evaluating AI/ML clinical trials in a standardized fashion. The Consolidated Standards of Reporting Trials–Artificial Intelligence provides general recommendations for reporting of AI clinical trials in medicine that have been endorsed by several scientific journals.[89] The Proposed Recommendations for Cardiovascular Imaging-Related Machine Learning Evaluation (PRIME) checklist provides best practice strategies to promote standardization and reduce bias more specifically related to cardiovascular imaging.[90] Guidelines for the use of AI for echocardiography and other specific modalities are likely to develop in the near future in light of the growing impact of AI and myriad challenges, including clinical trial reporting standardization, bias reduction, and the understanding of medicolegal consequences of using AI/ML in practice.[91] Adherence to reporting guidelines and sharing code and datasets when able would contribute to greater transparency, rigor, and reproducibility and acceleration research and application development in this area.[90,92–95]

In other areas of cardiovascular medicine, such as screening for atrial fibrillation or left ventricular dysfunction,[37,96–98] and in other specialties,[99] prospective cohort studies and clinical trials have helped form the foundation of the required evidence base for the scaling of these technologies. Similar studies in VHD will be essential to advancing the use of AI for improving outcomes for patients with VHD.

SUMMARY

VHD is a morbid condition in which AI has the potential to improve screening, diagnosis, phenomapping, and risk prediction. Currently, most of the research and applications remain relatively early in the development and implementation lifecycle. Future research should prioritize adherence to reporting guidelines, sharing code and datasets when able, external validation in diverse populations, measuring and reducing bias in algorithms, prospective evaluation in clinical trials, and development of systems for ongoing monitoring of model performance.

CLINICS CARE POINTS

- ML not only has the potential to improve the care of patients with VHD but also has pitfalls and limitations.
- ML approaches may in the future play an important role in the care of patients with VHD but AI-applications require rigorous testing, including prospective evaluation in clinical trials.

DISCLOSURE

F.S. Ahmad receives consulting fees from Pfizer and Livongo Teladoc outside of this study. C. Canning is an independent contractor at Tempus.

FUNDING

Dr Ahmad was supported by grants from the National Institutes of Health/National Heart, Lung, and Blood Institute (K23HL155970) and the American Heart Association (AHA number 856917).

REFERENCES

1. Marciniak A, Glover K, Sharma R. Cohort profile: prevalence of valvular heart disease in community patients with suspected heart failure in UK. BMJ Open 2017;7(1):e012240.
2. Philbin EF, DiSalvo TG. Prediction of hospital readmission for heart failure: development of a simple risk score based on administrative data. Rev Port Cardiol 1999;18(9):855–6.
3. Coffey S, Roberts-Thomson R, Brown A, et al. Global epidemiology of valvular heart disease. Nat Rev Cardiol 2021;18(12):853–64.
4. Chen J, Li W, Xiang M. Burden of valvular heart disease, 1990-2017: Results from the Global Burden of Disease Study 2017. J Glob Health 2020;10(2):20404.
5. Baumgartner H, Falk V, Bax JJ, et al. 2017 ESC/EACTS Guidelines for the management of valvular heart disease. Eur Heart J 2017;38(36):2739–91.

6. Carroll JD, Mack MJ, Vemulapalli S, et al. STS-ACC TVT Registry of Transcatheter Aortic Valve Replacement. J Am Coll Cardiol 2020;76(21):2492–516.

7. Mack M, Carroll JD, Thourani V, et al. Transcatheter Mitral Valve Therapy in the United States: A Report From the STS-ACC TVT Registry. J Am Coll Cardiol 2021;78(23):2326–53.

8. Goldberg YH, Ho E, Chau M, et al. Update on Transcatheter Tricuspid Valve Replacement Therapies. Front Cardiovasc Med 2021;8:619558.

9. Fam NP, von Bardeleben RS, Hensey M, et al. Transfemoral Transcatheter Tricuspid Valve Replacement With the EVOQUE System. JACC Cardiovasc Interv 2021;14(5):501–11.

10. Friedrich S, Groß S, König IR, et al. Applications of artificial intelligence/machine learning approaches in cardiovascular medicine: a systematic review with recommendations. Eur Heart J Digit Health 2021;2(3):424–36.

11. Beam AL, Kohane IS. Big Data and Machine Learning in Health Care. JAMA 2018;319(13): 1317–8.

12. Zhou J, Du M, Chang S, et al. Artificial intelligence in echocardiography: detection, functional evaluation, and disease diagnosis. Cardiovasc Ultrasound 2021;19(1):29.

13. Sermesant M, Delingette H, Cochet H, et al. Applications of artificial intelligence in cardiovascular imaging. Nat Rev Cardiol 2021;18(8):600–9.

14. Krishnan R, Rajpurkar P, Topol EJ. Self-supervised learning in medicine and healthcare. Nat Biomed Eng 2022. https://doi.org/10.1038/s41551-022-00914-1. Published online August 11.

15. Acosta JN, Falcone GJ, Rajpurkar P, et al. Multimodal biomedical AI. Nat Med 2022;28(9):1773–84.

16. Rajpurkar P, Chen E, Banerjee O, et al. AI in health and medicine. Nat Med 2022;28(1):31–8.

17. Ahmad FS, Luo Y, Wehbe RM, et al. Advances in Machine Learning Approaches to Heart Failure with Preserved Ejection Fraction. Heart Fail Clin 2022;18(2):287–300.

18. Otto CM, Nishimura RA, Bonow RO, et al. 2020 ACC/AHA Guideline for the Management of Patients With Valvular Heart Disease: A Report of the American College of Cardiology/American Heart Association Joint Committee on Clinical Practice Guidelines. Circulation 2021;143(5):e72–227.

19. Nkomo VT, Gardin JM, Skelton TN, et al. Burden of valvular heart diseases: a population-based study. Lancet 2006;368(9540):1005–11.

20. Alexander KM, Orav J, Singh A, et al. Geographic Disparities in Reported US Amyloidosis Mortality From 1979 to 2015: Potential Underdetection of Cardiac Amyloidosis. JAMA Cardiol 2018;3(9):865–70.

21. d'Arcy JL, Coffey S, Loudon MA, et al. Large-scale community echocardiographic screening reveals a major burden of undiagnosed valvular heart disease in older people: the OxVALVE Population Cohort. Eur Heart J. Published online 2016. Available at: https://academic.oup.com/eurheartj/article-abstract/37/47/3515/2844994.

22. Maron MS, Hellawell JL, Lucove JC, et al. Occurrence of Clinically Diagnosed Hypertrophic Cardiomyopathy in the United States. Am J Cardiol 2016; 117(10):1651–4.

23. Kang DH, Park SJ, Lee SA, et al. Early Surgery or Conservative Care for Asymptomatic Aortic Stenosis. N Engl J Med 2020;382(2):111–9.

24. Carabello BA. Aortic Valve Replacement Should Be Operated on Before Symptom Onset. Circulation 2012;126(1):112–7.

25. Ross J Jr, Braunwald E. Aortic stenosis. Circulation 1968;38(1 Suppl):61–7.

26. Cheitlin MD, Gertz EW, Brundage BH, et al. Rate of progression of severity of valvular aortic stenosis in the adult. Am Heart J 1979;98(6):689–700.

27. Curtis JP, Sokol SI, Wang Y, et al. The association of left ventricular ejection fraction, mortality, and cause of death in stable outpatients with heart failure. J Am Coll Cardiol 2003;42(4):736–42.

28. Dobrow RJ, Calatayud JB, Abraham S, et al. A study of physician variation in heart-sound interpretation. Med Ann Dist Columbia 1964;33:305–8.

29. Etchells E, Bell C, Robb K. Does This Patient Have an Abnormal Systolic Murmur? JAMA 1997;277(7): 564–71.

30. Clifford GD, Liu C, Moody B, et al. Classification of normal/abnormal heart sound recordings: The PhysioNet/Computing in Cardiology Challenge 2016. In: 2016 computing in cardiology conference (CinC). 2016. p. 609–12.

31. Clifford GD, Liu C, Moody B, et al. Recent advances in heart sound analysis. Physiol Meas 2017;38(8): E10–25.

32. Swarup S, Makaryus AN. Digital stethoscope: technology update. Med Devices 2018;11:29–36.

33. Chorba JS, Shapiro AM, Le L, et al. Deep Learning Algorithm for Automated Cardiac Murmur Detection via a Digital Stethoscope Platform. J Am Heart Assoc 2021;10(9):e019905.

34. Carabello BA. Transcatheter aortic-valve implantation for aortic stenosis in patients who cannot undergo surgery. Curr Cardiol Rep 2011;13(3): 173–4.

35. Ben-Dor I, Pichard AD, Gonzalez MA, et al. Correlates and causes of death in patients with severe symptomatic aortic stenosis who are not eligible to participate in a clinical trial of transcatheter aortic valve implantation. Circulation 2010;122(11 Suppl): S37–42.

36. Kwon JM, Lee SY, Jeon KH, et al. Deep Learning-Based Algorithm for Detecting Aortic Stenosis Using Electrocardiography. J Am Heart Assoc 2020;9(7): e014717.

37. Cohen-Shelly M, Attia ZI, Friedman PA, et al. Electro-cardiogram screening for aortic valve stenosis using artificial intelligence. Eur Heart J 2021;42(30): 2885–96.

38. Ghassemi M, Oakden-Rayner L, Beam AL. The false hope of current approaches to explainable artificial intelligence in health care. Lancet Digit Health 2021;3(11):e745–50.

39. Saporta A, Gui X, Agrawal A, et al. Benchmarking saliency methods for chest X-ray interpretation. Nat Mach Intell 2022;4(10):867–78.

40. Ulloa-Cerna AE, Jing L, Pfeifer JM, et al. rECHOm-mend: An ECG-Based Machine Learning Approach for Identifying Patients at Increased Risk of Undiag-nosed Structural Heart Disease Detectable by Echocardiography. Circulation 2022;146(1):36–47.

41. Papolos A, Narula J, Bavishi C, et al. Hospital Use of Echocardiography: Insights From the Nationwide Inpa-tient Sample. J Am Coll Cardiol 2016;67(5):502–11.

42. Douglas PS, Khandheria B, Stainback RF, et al. ACCF/ASE/ACEP/AHA/ASNC/SCAI/SCCT/SCMR 2008 appropriateness criteria for stress echocardi-ography: a report of the American College of Cardi-ology Foundation Appropriateness Criteria Task Force, American Society of Echocardiography, American College of Emergency Physicians, Amer-ican Heart Association, American Society of Nuclear Cardiology, Society for Cardiovascular Angiography and Interventions, Society of Cardiovascular Computed Tomography, and Society for Cardiovas-cular Magnetic Resonance endorsed by the Heart Rhythm Society and the Society of Critical Care Medicine. J Am Coll Cardiol 2008;51(11):1127–47.

43. Matulevicius SA, Rohatgi A, Das SR, et al. Appro-priate use and clinical impact of transthoracic echo-cardiography. JAMA Intern Med 2013;173(17): 1600–7.

44. Zhang J, Gajjala S, Agrawal P, et al. Fully automated echocardiogram interpretation in clinical practice. Circulation 2018;138(16):1623–35.

45. Ghorbani A, Ouyang D, Abid A, et al. Deep Learning Interpretation of Echocardiograms. doi:10.1101/681676.

46. Tromp J, Bauer D, Claggett BL, et al. A formal vali-dation of a deep learning-based automated work-flow for the interpretation of the echocardiogram. Nat Commun 2022;13(1):6776.

47. Ouyang D, He B, Ghorbani A, et al. Video-based AI for beat-to-beat assessment of cardiac function. Na-ture 2020;580(7802):252–6. https://doi.org/10.1038/s41586-020-2145-8.

48. Madani A, Arnaout R, Mofrad M, et al. Fast and ac-curate view classification of echocardiograms using deep learning. NPJ Digit Med 2018;1. https://doi.org/10.1038/s41746-017-0013-1.

49. Abdi AH, Luong C, Tsang T, et al. Automatic Quality Assessment of Echocardiograms Using Convolutional

Neural Networks: Feasibility on the Apical Four-Chamber View. IEEE Trans Med Imaging 2017;36(6): 1221–30.

50. Asch FM, Poilvert N, Abraham T, et al. Automated Echocardiographic Quantification of Left Ventricular Ejection Fraction Without Volume Measurements Us-ing a Machine Learning Algorithm Mimicking a Hu-man Expert. Circ Cardiovasc Imaging 2019;12(9): e009303.

51. Diller GP, Babu-Narayan S, Li W, et al. Utility of ma-chine learning algorithms in assessing patients with a systemic right ventricle. Eur Heart J Cardiovasc Imaging 2019;20(8):925–31.

52. Goto S, Mahara K, Beussink-Nelson L, et al. Artificial intelligence-enabled fully automated detection of cardiac amyloidosis using electrocardiograms and echocardiograms. Nat Commun 2021;12(1):2726.

53. Goto S, Solanki D, John JE, et al. Multinational Federated Learning Approach to Train ECG and Echocardiogram Models for Hypertrophic Cardio-myopathy Detection. Circulation 2022;146(10): 755–69.

54. Duffy G, Cheng PP, Yuan N, et al. High-Throughput Precision Phenotyping of Left Ventricular Hypertro-phy With Cardiovascular Deep Learning. JAMA Car-diol 2022;7(4):386–95.

55. Soto JT, Weston Hughes J, Sanchez PA, et al. Multi-modal deep learning enhances diagnostic precision in left ventricular hypertrophy. Eur Heart J Digit Health 2022;3(3):380–9.

56. Yang Feifei, Chen Xiaotian, Lin Xixiang, et al. Auto-mated Analysis of Doppler Echocardiographic Videos as a Screening Tool for Valvular Heart Dis-eases. JACC Cardiovasc Imaging 2022;15(4): 551–63.

57. Sengupta Partho P, Shrestha S, Kagiyama N, et al. A Machine-Learning Framework to Identify Distinct Phenotypes of Aortic Stenosis Severity. JACC Cardi-ovasc Imaging 2021;14(9):1707–20.

58. Poilvert N, Goldstein S, Lang RM, et al. Abstract 14356: Machine Learning for Detection of Presence and Severity of Aortic Stenosis From B-mode Ultra-sound Images: Results of a Blinded Clinical Trial. Circulation 2022;146(Suppl_1):A14356.

59. Playford D, Bordin E, Mohamad R, et al. Enhanced Diagnosis of Severe Aortic Stenosis Using Artificial Intelligence: A Proof-of-Concept Study of 530,871 Echocardiograms. JACC Cardiovasc Imaging 2020;13(4):1087–90.

60. Narang A, Bae R, Hong H, et al. Utility of a Deep-Learning Algorithm to Guide Novices to Acquire Echocardiograms for Limited Diagnostic Use. JAMA Cardiol 2021;6(6):624–32.

61. Solomon MD, Tabada G, Allen A, et al. Large-scale identification of aortic stenosis and its severity using natural language processing on electronic health re-cords. Cardiovasc Digit Health J 2021;2(3):156–63.

62. Strom JB, Xu J, Sun T, et al. Characterizing the Accuracy of International Classification of Diseases, Tenth Revision Administrative Claims for Aortic Valve Disease. Circulation 2022;15(10). https://doi.org/10.1161/circoutcomes.122.009162.

63. Thomas JD, Petrescu OM, Moualla SK, et al. Artificial intelligence to assist physicians in identifying patients with severe aortic stenosis. Intelligence-Based Medicine 2022;6:100059.

64. Allen LA, Venechuk G, McIlvennan CK, et al. An Electronically Delivered Patient-Activation Tool for Intensification of Medications for Chronic Heart Failure With Reduced Ejection Fraction: The EPIC-HF Trial. Circulation 2021;143(5):427–37.

65. Baljash Cheema, Kannan Mutharasan R, Sharma Aditya, et al. Augmented Intelligence to Identify Patients With Advanced Heart Failure in an Integrated Health System. JACC (J Am Coll Cardiol): Advances 2022;1(4):1–11.

66. Wells PS, Anderson DR, Rodger M, et al. Excluding pulmonary embolism at the bedside without diagnostic imaging: management of patients with suspected pulmonary embolism presenting to the emergency department by using a simple clinical model and d-dimer. Ann Intern Med 2001;135(2):98–107.

67. Seymour CW, Liu VX, Iwashyna TJ, et al. Assessment of Clinical Criteria for Sepsis: For the Third International Consensus Definitions for Sepsis and Septic Shock (Sepsis-3). JAMA 2016;315(8): 762–74.

68. Clavel MA, Magne J, Pibarot P. Low-gradient aortic stenosis. Eur Heart J 2016;37(34):2645–57.

69. Namasivayam M, Myers PD, Guttag JV, et al. Predicting outcomes in patients with aortic stenosis using machine learning: the Aortic Stenosis Risk (ASteRisk) score. Open Heart 2022;9(1). https://doi.org/10.1136/openhrt-2022-001990.

70. Lee SP, Lee W, Lee JM, et al. Assessment of diffuse myocardial fibrosis by using MR imaging in asymptomatic patients with aortic stenosis. Radiology 2015;274(2):359–69.

71. Kwak S, Everett RJ, Treibel TA, et al. Markers of Myocardial Damage Predict Mortality in Patients With Aortic Stenosis. J Am Coll Cardiol 2021;78(6): 545–58.

72. Bohbot Y, Raitière O, Guignant P, et al. Unsupervised clustering of patients with severe aortic stenosis: A myocardial continuum. Arch Cardiovasc Dis. Published online September 2022;29. https://doi.org/10.1016/j.acvd.2022.06.007.

73. Lachmann M, Rippen E, Schuster T, et al. Subphenotyping of Patients With Aortic Stenosis by Unsupervised Agglomerative Clustering of Echocardiographic and Hemodynamic Data. JACC Cardiovasc Interv 2021; 14(19):2127–40.

74. Kwak S, Lee Y, Ko T, et al. Unsupervised Cluster Analysis of Patients With Aortic Stenosis Reveals Distinct Population With Different Phenotypes and Outcomes. Circ Cardiovasc Imaging 2020;13(5): e009707.

75. Ouyang D, Thomas JD. Characterizing Mitral Regurgitation With Precision Phenotyping and Unsupervised Learning. JACC Cardiovasc Imaging 2021; 14(12):2301–2.

76. Bartko PE, Heitzinger G, Spinka G, et al. Principal Morphomic and Functional Components of Secondary Mitral Regurgitation. JACC Cardiovasc Imaging 2021;14(12):2288–300.

77. Stone GW, Lindenfeld J, Abraham WT, et al. Transcatheter Mitral-Valve Repair in Patients with Heart Failure. N Engl J Med 2018;379(24):2307–18.

78. Obadia JF, Messika-Zeitoun D, Leurent G, et al. Percutaneous Repair or Medical Treatment for Secondary Mitral Regurgitation. N Engl J Med 2018; 379(24):2297–306.

79. Kline A, Wang H, Li Y, et al. Multimodal machine learning in precision health: A scoping review. NPJ Digit Med 2022;5(1):171.

80. OpenAI. ChatGPT. Optimizing Language Models for Dialogue. OpenAI 2022. Available at: https://openai.com/blog/chatgpt/. Accessed February 25, 2023.

81. Benjamens S, Dhunnoo P, Meskó B. The state of artificial intelligence-based FDA-approved medical devices and algorithms: an online database. NPJ Digit Med 2020;3:118.

82. Li RC, Asch SM, Shah NH. Developing a delivery science for artificial intelligence in healthcare. NPJ Digit Med 2020;3:107.

83. Marwaha JS, Landman AB, Brat GA, et al. Deploying digital health tools within large, complex health systems: key considerations for adoption and implementation. NPJ Digit Med 2022;5(1):13.

84. Finlayson SG, Subbaswamy A, Singh K, et al. The Clinician and Dataset Shift in Artificial Intelligence. N Engl J Med 2021;385(3):283–6.

85. Gianfrancesco MA, Tamang S, Yazdany J, et al. Potential Biases in Machine Learning Algorithms Using Electronic Health Record Data. JAMA Intern Med 2018;178(11):1544–7.

86. Hajian S, Bonchi F, Castillo C. Algorithmic Bias: From Discrimination Discovery to Fairness-aware Data Mining. In: Proceedings of the 22nd ACM SIGKDD international conference on knowledge discovery and data mining. KDD '16. Association for Computing Machinery; 2016. p. 2125–6.

87. Larrazabal AJ, Nieto N, Peterson V, et al. Gender imbalance in medical imaging datasets produces biased classifiers for computer-aided diagnosis. Proc Natl Acad Sci U S A 2020;117(23):12592–4.

88. Obermeyer Z, Powers B, Vogeli C, et al. Dissecting racial bias in an algorithm used to manage the health of populations. Science 2019;366(6464):447–53.

89. Liu X, Cruz Rivera S, Moher D, et al, CONSORT-AI Working Group. Reporting guidelines for clinical trial

reports for interventions involving artificial intelligence: the CONSORT-AI extension. Nat Med 2020; 26(9):1364–74.

90. Sengupta PP, Shrestha S, Berthon B, et al. Proposed Requirements for Cardiovascular Imaging-Related Machine Learning Evaluation (PRIME): A Checklist: Reviewed by the American College of Cardiology Healthcare Innovation Council. JACC Cardiovasc Imaging 2020;13(9):2017–35.

91. Tseng AS, Lopez-Jimenez F, Pellikka PA. Future Guidelines for Artificial Intelligence in Echocardiography. J Am Soc Echocardiogr 2022;35(8): 878–82.

92. Collins GS, Dhiman P, Andaur Navarro CL, et al. Protocol for development of a reporting guideline (TRIPOD-AI) and risk of bias tool (PROBAST-AI) for diagnostic and prognostic prediction model studies based on artificial intelligence. BMJ Open 2021; 11(7):e048008.

93. Vasey B, Nagendran M, Campbell B, et al. Reporting guideline for the early-stage clinical evaluation of decision support systems driven by artificial intelligence: DECIDE-AI. Nat Med 2022;28(5):924–33.

94. Liu Y, Chen PHC, Krause J, et al. How to Read Articles That Use Machine Learning: Users' Guides to the Medical Literature. JAMA 2019;322(18): 1806–16.

95. Stevens LM, Mortazavi BJ, Deo RC, et al. Recommendations for Reporting Machine Learning Analyses in Clinical Research. Circ Cardiovasc Qual Outcomes 2020;13(10):e006556.

96. Perez MV, Mahaffey KW, Hedlin H, et al. Large-Scale Assessment of a Smartwatch to Identify Atrial Fibrillation. N Engl J Med 2019;381(20):1909–17.

97. Attia ZI, Harmon DM, Dugan J, et al. Prospective evaluation of smartwatch-enabled detection of left ventricular dysfunction. Nat Med 2022;28(12):2497–503.

98. Yao X, Rushlow DR, Inselman JW, et al. Artificial intelligence-enabled electrocardiograms for identification of patients with low ejection fraction: a pragmatic, randomized clinical trial. Nat Med 2021;27(5):815–9.

99. Plana D, Shung DL, Grimshaw AA, et al. Randomized Clinical Trials of Machine Learning Interventions in Health Care: A Systematic Review. JAMA Netw Open 2022;5(9):e2233946.

Moving?

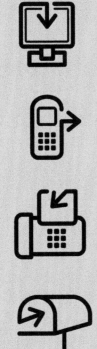

Make sure your subscription moves with you!

To notify us of your new address, find your **Clinics Account Number** (located on your mailing label above your name), and contact customer service at:

Email: journalscustomerservice-usa@elsevier.com

800-654-2452 (subscribers in the U.S. & Canada)
314-447-8871 (subscribers outside of the U.S. & Canada)

Fax number: 314-447-8029

Elsevier Health Sciences Division
Subscription Customer Service
3251 Riverport Lane
Maryland Heights, MO 63043

Printed and bound by CPI Group (UK) Ltd, Croydon, CR0 4YY

03/10/2024

01040363-0011